Get UP!

Defy Aging with Movement

Get UP!

Defy Aging with Movement

Nancy Alexander, PT

ISBN: 978-1-7359183-0-3 (sc)

ISBN: 978-1-7359183-1-0 (e)

Library of Congress Control Number: 2020925005

Author photos: Courtesy of Steve Chesler, Chesler Photography

Publisher: Living Well Now LLC, PO Box 3373, Apollo Beach, Florida 33572

Website: www.prosolutions55.com

Author Contact: livewellnow55@gmail.com

Dedication

I humbly dedicate this book to all my current and former patients and clients. For the past 25 years, you allowed me the opportunity to offer you hope and guidance in your time of need. You taught me so much. Thank you for inspiring me.

Contents

Acknowledgments

Thank you to the physical therapists, occupational therapists, speech therapists, athletic trainers, PT assistants, and rehab aides I've had the pleasure to work with over so many years. I am honored to still know many of you as friends today. Thank you to the teams of physicians, nurses, and other allied health professionals who joined me in the interest of helping our patients recover and thrive. I learned so much from all of you–too much to justly describe here. And in turn, you helped our patients, too. Cheers to you.

Thank you to my editor, project manager, and mentor Judith Shenouda. You have inspired me since we first met. You are smart, kind, and courageous. After a brief meeting, we stayed connected and our relationship grew. Your encouragement and openness to collaborate together on many projects over the years are gestures I will always cherish. Here's to always learning and growing.

Thank you, Jennifer Alexander, for again having my back and making sure this book was finished in a timely manner. Accountability agreements work, and accountability partners are incredibly valuable. You, Jennifer, are that and much more. You are beautiful in every way. Thank you.

Thank you to those featured in my stories in this book. You are examples of grit, determination, and persistence few possess. You have inspired me more than you will ever know. And now, with this book, you will inspire and teach so many more. Thank you.

Thank you to my late mother and father, Jean and Jim Alexander, who showed me love endlessly and told me I could do whatever I wanted with my life. Because of you, I am.

Last but not least, thank you, Ron. Thanks for embracing my crazy dreams and believing in me. Your confidence in me and your support of me mean the world to me. It's pretty cool when your "What if's?" become, "Wow, that was awesome!"

Dream on and keep moving.

Praise for Get UP! Defy Aging with Movement

"I really enjoyed reading Nancy's perspective on the importance of moving to build strength, confidence and maintaining your independence. Her stories about clients and their success were inspiring. A small consistent effort can make a large impact on your health and lifestyle. No fancy equipment needed, just a desire to start a new chapter."

Amy Hoffman
Former Business Executive and Entrepreneur

"Nancy's inspiration shines through as she provides a comprehensive resource to help improve your quality of life. Her thoughtful and supportive approach will motivate you to get up and get moving."

J.J. Mowder-Tinney PT, PhD, NCS, CEEAA,
C/NDT, CSRS
Physical Therapist, Professor, and Speaker

"*Get UP! Defy Aging with Movement* is an easy read that made me want to do just that…GET UP. I consider myself to be pretty active, but Nancy Alexander has the experience and talent that made me see that I can always do more. It's a great how-to manual for building a simple plan for yourself, so you can succeed at better mobility and long-term health."

Laurie O'Shaughnessy
Retired CEO-Greater Canandaigua Family YMCA

"Nancy Alexander is an engaging, encouraging, and passionate clinician and coach. Whether in a class, in post-op therapy, or in an individual training session, Nancy's depth of knowledge and genuine delight in her clients are evident the first hour one spends with her. That same friendly, approachable voice is evident on every page of *Get UP! Defy Aging with Movement*. Moreover, it is her years of experience and thorough research that make the book such a worthwhile resource. Nancy is surely intent upon *moving* us into the most healthy and productive season of our lives."

Linda Sage-Fenti
Retired Educator and Active Adult

Introduction

So many people think it's natural for your activity to decline as you age. Are you one of them? Truth is, many of you are physically capable of moving, but you choose not to move. Movement as you age is more important than at any other time in your history. To enjoy a high quality of life, you must move and continue to move.

Usually in their 50s, many adults stop doing the activities they used to do and that they enjoyed. Maybe it's due to fear of injury or maybe your performance doesn't match the expectation. Maybe you hurt. Maybe you've told yourself you are too old to even try. Do you accept it? Is this a fact? Or is it merely an opinion? Is it your opinion?

As a licensed physical therapist (PT) and certified fitness professional for over 25 years, I have seen what movement can do for a body. I have also seen what little to no movement has done for a body. I have seen what a fixed mindset about activity and exercise can do to someone. Mobility is one of the most important aspects of living well over 50. You have complete control over your movement and you must fiercely protect it. Move this up on your priority list. If you want your next years to be your best years, it starts with movement.

You must realize this, act, and act now to stop this progression. Why? Because you can–and because your life depends on it. Research repeatedly shows the benefits of movement and exercise on our bodies and our quality of life. In this book, I'll highlight the latest research and its impact. I'll share stories of inspiration throughout my years as a PT and fitness professional.

It's true this journey is part physical and part mental. Okay, maybe a lot mental. We'll talk more about that in this book. In fact, I have a whole chapter devoted to it. To ignore this aspect of movement would be a disservice. Don't be fooled by what you think are your limitations. Challenge your beliefs and expectations. You don't always know what you can or cannot do.

Maybe you're wondering, "Will I hurt myself more?" Maybe you're asking yourself, "Where do I start?" These are all valid questions. This book provides guidelines to help you find these answers. As a PT, I'm trained to start you in a safe place that is effective for you.

Put your mind to work here because, in reality, you get what you think about. Your mind is incredibly powerful. Harness its power first by not complaining, blaming others, or justifying your current situation. This is a no judgment zone. Own where you are (your starting point) and move on. We all have our own starting points. What matters is that you choose not to dwell on what you can't do. There is always something you can do. Focus on that. Your starting point is starting to look better, isn't it?

I'm going to meet this next concept head on. What is movement? What is exercise? Movement is just that—your body or part of it moves or changes position. It's a physiological miracle. Even so, I have learned over the years that the term *exercise* is a real turnoff for some folks. "I don't exercise," some say. "I don't like to exercise," they add. But do you move? Of course, you move.

Exercise is purposeful movement. I could dress up exercise so you don't recognize it as such. I'll put a big overcoat on it with a hat, glasses, and a moustache. And then I'll ask you to walk up the stairs. Do you view that as exercise or movement? Regardless of your label, some see it as critical because the only bathroom is upstairs. You moved to get there, right? It's really both exercise and movement.

I've met many who profess not to like exercise. If that is the case, please read on and open your mind to think of exercise as purposeful movement. Think of it as using your muscles, your joints, and your skeletal system to make something purposeful happen. Your body is a miracle.

Walking is purposeful movement, especially when you're in the grocery store buying food for your family. Reaching and lifting in the kitchen are purposeful when it comes time to prepare a meal. Reaching down to your feet is purposeful if you want to dress in the morning. For the purpose of this book, let's think movement. Movement is pure, movement is natural, movement is how we live a life. Movement is how we have fun. Exercise is a type of movement. Please stay with me here. Open your mind to movement.

What are your goals? They are your foundation and you'll have the opportunity to define these more as part of this book. In fact, you will build your own movement plan right here. By the end of this book, you will have an actionable plan with realistic next steps that will take you to a better life. I will let you in on how a PT develops a plan of care for each patient that is designed to target specific needs. Then, I'll lead you through each component and modify it to help you strategically develop your own plan. Chapters 2, 5, 8, and 12 all end with an activity that will lead you through the thought process required to create this plan. Feel free to use your own journal or use the Notes section at the back of this book to start this process. I'm so excited to see where your plan will take you.

Everyone's needs and desires are different. Maybe you've used a walker for years after an illness but want to learn to walk with less of a device or maybe even without a device. This was a goal of one of my more recent clients. And guess what? Goal achieved. I am so proud of this man's motivation and accomplishments. By the way, he did this at age 80. Maybe you want to go on that bucket list trip of a lifetime but fear your mobility compromises you. Maybe you want to keep up with your active husband or wife. Maybe you want the stamina to play with your grandkids. Maybe you're watching your friends have all kinds of fun learning how to play pickleball and now you want to try. Maybe you want to try riding your bicycle a couple of days per week to stay in shape. Maybe you want to play golf again. It's been years since you've played, but you really want to get back out there. Maybe you want to enjoy the 19th hole with your friends and share stories that make you laugh. Sometimes, that's the best part of golf or any sport, right? Movement is a gateway to fellowship.

I want you to move because you want to move, because you know the benefits first hand. I don't want you to move because someone else wants you to move. Maybe your daughter hounds you to exercise and it's a real turnoff. Maybe your husband complains you won't join him in the gym. Maybe you try to exercise to appease them, but in the end, it typically doesn't last long and the old habits return. Let's turn this around. Don't think about what they want for you. What do you want? This is a rightful focus, a great place to start, and it has staying power.

My role as a PT is that of a professional educator. To that end, I discuss the aging process in Chapters 3 and 4. I guess you can say these chapters go together. There are changes the body goes through as we age that I discuss in Chapter 3. Each body system is identified and I share how aging impacts each one. Then, in Chapter 4, I describe how movement and exercise help reverse the aging process. Again, this is organized by body system. Movement makes miracles happen.

My role as an author is that of a story teller. In this book, you'll find stories and lessons I've learned from some of the thousands of patients I've treated over the years. Many of my patients and clients overcame extreme obstacles to recover from their injury or illness. I can't wait for you to meet these amazing individuals here. Don't worry. Confidentiality reigns and all names have been changed except for very few who gave their expressed permission. I hope they inspire you as much as they've inspired me. It was a privilege to be a part of each one of their lives.

You would need a prescription from your physician for PT to learn a lot of what is in this book. I freely offer it to you here because I want to help you feel better, move better, and live better. I want you to make your next years your best years.

This is the promise I made in memory of my dear father, Jim Alexander. My father participated in sports most of his life and played ice hockey and softball into his 60s. I learned to appreciate the joys of an active life from him, and his inspiration has carried me far in my life. Maybe you've met my father reading my first book, *An Unlikely Gift: Finding Inspiration Caring for My Father with Dementia*. I adored him and I wanted to be like him. I am in many ways. I value movement, too, and continue to participate in multiple sports and plan to do so as long as I can. It doesn't just happen. We need to manage our bodies, and continued movement is key. I'm doing it, too. In this book, you'll learn why movement matters and discover how you can continue to move, too.

That's right, I'll show you how to get started. Later in this book, I offer specific exercises and activities successfully used by thousands of my patients to help get you started and keep you moving. Be safe and always consult with your physician prior to starting any new exercise program, including this one.

I want to give you the tools to get moving again. If you are already active, great. I hope to give you some ideas to progress and add a little variety to your moves. I hope to make your movement more meaningful. I want you to live a good life. I want to help you return to those activities you enjoy. I want to help you spend more time with family and friends. I want to help you take your health to the next level where you can survive and even thrive whatever your environment throws your way. All of this is my dream for you.

Does your pain continue? Do you miss doing the things you enjoy? Remember this, whatever your age or fitness level, you cannot keep doing the same things and expect a different result. That's insanity. Movement can help you return to the activities you enjoy. Movement can help you live longer, too. Research backs that up. More importantly perhaps, movement can help your next years be your best years. You can live longer while also enjoying a good quality of life. Magic? No. It's about movement.

There is way too much living to do. Your future starts now. So, let's get moving.

Chapter 1 Movement Is Medicine

Movement is your magic pill. Movement is your fountain of youth. Movement can save your life. Never give up

That's what my former client Bonnie would tell you. At age 60 she experienced what she describes as her defining moment. It was a horrendous car accident that few could survive. She did survive and because she did, she lives with a passion to be active and healthy and encourages others to do the same.

She still remembers it well. It was in 2006 and she recalls she had a new grand-daughter. She was coming home from her hairdresser. She was driving up a hill and then lost consciousness. She drifted into the other lane where she crashed into another vehicle. "They say the combined effective speed was about 80 mph," said Bonnie. She regained consciousness briefly after the collision when they were cutting the car apart to get her out. It had collapsed around her. She opened her eyes, and she saw her arms up in the air. Her right arm had an obvious open forearm fracture with a lot of exposed bone. She remembers the ambulance taking her to the hospital. She had multiple fractures—both bones at her right forearm, every rib, and sternum. She also had a separation of the left clavicle at her sternum. In addition, she had a collapsed lung. The most serious injury was a transecting aorta (otherwise known as an aortic rupture), the result of the abrupt deceleration from speed to stop. Fortunately, it was slow to develop and was repaired with a stent. This was the first time a stent was used for an accident repair and was 100 percent successful. Bonnie is a walking miracle.

Bonnie said she drew strength from her family and friends. "I had some very dark times," she said. Recovery was complicated by developing reflex sympathetic dystrophy (RSD) syndrome, which is a complex and chronic regional pain syndrome that affects limbs after injury, surgery, a stroke, or heart attack. She had to have injections to get through the pain of being stretched and ranged as part of her rehabilitation. There was emotional pain, too. Bonnie learned the other driver survived and was grateful for that. "That haunted me," she said.

"So many people give up–it's easy to do," Bonnie added. "The medical professionals who worked with me said I would never be able to rotate my right forearm again. I can. Their prognosis made me more determined." Since her accident, Bonnie has had both her knees replaced due to arthritis. She has also had a shoulder replacement and hip replacement.

"I didn't give up then and I don't want to give up now," Bonnie said. "There's so much living yet to do. Life is great as long as I can be active."

Bonnie admits that she got very depressed during the long recovery and enforced inactivity. To go from being very active to sitting in a recliner 24/7 was incredibly depressing for her. "I got the idea that I had to let the bad feelings out from time to time or go crazy," Bonnie said. "I started having what I called pity parties. I would look at the clock and say to myself, You've got 10 minutes, then you're done. Scream, cry, do whatever you want, then go back to being positive and upbeat. "Make sure you are alone when you do this," Bonnie added with a half-smile. Bonnie wants to remind others that they are human. "You're going to feel sorry for yourself. But you also need to set limits for this."

More importantly, Bonnie focuses on what she can do. Among her many interests and activities, Bonnie loves to travel. Bonnie has been active for years with equestrian events and is a would-be competitive dressage rider. She bikes and enjoys yoga and Pilates classes. She is a certified Alpine Level 2 ski instructor. She is also a senior level ski patroller. She ran a marathon at age 52 in Dublin, Ireland, which she said was one of the biggest challenges she has ever done.

Bonnie said her recovery from her accident lasted about one year and that the only limitation from it is that she can't completely straighten her fourth finger on her right hand. That is remarkable by any standard. "If I had not been in such good shape when it happened, I was told I may not have survived," Bonnie said.

"Never give up. Keep moving. Find mental and physical challenges. Find challenges that are achievable and meaningful," she added. "Face your struggles head on." Movement saved Bonnie's life. Movement has defined mine.

I graduated high school in 1979. Title IX legislation passed in 1972. Title IX states that, "No person in the United States shall, on the basis of sex, be excluded from participation in, be denied the benefits of, or be subjected to discrimination under any education program or activity receiving Federal financial assistance." (U.S. Department of Education, Title IX and Sex Discrimination) Bless Title IX. Girls and women now had opportunities to play sports like never before. Schools and colleges had to more evenly offer sports clubs and teams to boys and girls. Participation in sports for girls exploded. Girls moved like never before.

I learned how to move with a purpose while playing sports. Ice hockey and sports changed me. Once a very shy girl, sports gave me an avenue to grow and learn about myself. I was a very different girl on the ice than off. I learned to like that girl on the ice and decided to bring that girl with me to other areas of my life. I learned how to be a better person, a better daughter, a better friend, and a better teammate. All thanks to sports and especially ice hockey. All thanks to movement.

I have participated in other sports in my life, too such as skiing, softball, volleyball, pickleball, soccer, and golf. I played hard and had my share of injuries, just like many of you. I was a patient in physical therapy for the summer after my sophomore year when I hurt my low back playing college hockey at SUNY College at Oswego. I had these episodes when my back would just give out. One slight lean forward and I was in intense pain and dropped to the floor, or ice if I was playing at the time. I didn't play college hockey after that year. Practicing or playing a game almost every day of the week was just too painful. I was advised by my physician to give up playing hockey at that time. It was then he told me that if I didn't give up playing hockey, I may not be able to have children one day. I have to say I didn't understand this. Quite frankly, I didn't believe him. He offered no rational reason for this. He just said it. Can it be this bad? I thought.

He didn't realize it, but he made me more determined to play than ever. I worked hard and focused on restoring flexibility and strengthening my back and my core. Three years later I was playing again.

Years later I had imaging performed on my back. and I have two torn discs in my lumbar spine that have since scarred over. I have arthritis and disc desiccation at multiple levels in my lumbar spine. Disc desiccation is one of the most common features of degenerative disc disease. It refers to dehydration of the discs. These discs are much squattier and darker on x-ray than other, healthier discs. I also have spondylolisthesis at L4 and L5. This means one vertebra is permanently misaligned and more forward than the one below it. I could have been born with this, but I just don't know. It is what it is.

Later in my hockey career, I sustained a compression fracture at my thoracic spine (T6) and fractured two ribs. I separated my right sternoclavicular joint (the joint at my sternum and collar bone). It continues to jut forward and always will. I also have stenosis at my neck, which occasionally flares up with pain and altered sensation at my right arm. My spine is a mess, but I manage it and will manage it for the rest of my life. And I wouldn't trade a thing. I would do it all again in a heartbeat.

I have physical therapy to thank for getting me back on the ice, enjoying a game I love. When my physician warned me about not being able to have children, I decided to ask him if I could go to physical therapy. The athletic trainers at SUNY Oswego told me that I would benefit from it. I had to ask for it, but he obliged and I decided to have therapy at the same clinic used by members of the New York Islanders, the professional hockey team on Long Island where I lived. They know hockey players, right?

My PT was a miracle worker. I attended therapy twice a week that summer, and it helped me more than I can describe. I was not able to play any further in college, but later I played in women's recreational leagues for over 32 years. That's right, 32 years. You see I learned a lot about my body in therapy and learned to keep it as flexible and strong as I could. I learned to listen to my body better and know when I was becoming vulnerable.

Title IX brought me movement, and movement brought me sports. Movement brought me hockey that I shared with my dear father for over 40 years. Movement brought me all kinds of amazing people to my life. Many are still my friends today. Movement brought me health. It brought me fun. Movement brought me happiness. Movement brought me confidence as a teenage girl who honestly didn't have much from the start. Movement brought me a wonderful career that continues today. Movement brought me thousands of patients, which led to glorious friendships. Movement even brought me my husband. Don't worry. This was not scandalous. But that is how we met. We dated after he was discharged. The rest is history as they say.

Movement Is life

We'll be talking about all different kinds of movement in this book. Movement can range from normal daily activities to participation in a sport. Movement can include an exercise routine you created to help keep you fit and healthy. If you're having trouble trying to move more or beginning an exercise plan and then following through, you're not alone. Many of us struggle getting out of the sedentary rut, despite our best intentions.

There are many great reasons to exercise–from improving energy, mood, sleep, and health to reducing anxiety, stress, and depression. And exercise instruction and workout plans are everywhere it seems, just a click away. But if knowing how and why to exercise were enough, we'd all be in shape. Making exercise a habit takes more–you need the right mindset and a smart approach.

While practical concerns like a busy schedule or poor health can make exercise more challenging, for most of us, the biggest barriers are mental. Maybe it's a lack of self-confidence that keeps you from taking positive steps, or your motivation quickly flames out, or you get easily discouraged and give up. We've all been there at some point. Whatever your age or fitness level–even if you've never exercised a day in your life–there are steps you can take to make exercise less intimidating and painful and more fun and instinctive.

Ditch the all-or-nothing attitude. You don't have to spend hours in a gym or force yourself into monotonous or painful activities you hate to experience the physical and emotional benefits of exercise. A little exercise is better than nothing. In fact, adding just modest amounts of physical activity to your weekly routine can have a profound effect on your mental and emotional health.

Be kind to yourself. Research shows that self-compassion increases the likelihood that you'll succeed in any given endeavor. So, don't beat yourself up about your body, your current fitness level, or your supposed lack of willpower. All that will do is demotivate you. Instead, look at your past mistakes and unhealthy choices as opportunities to learn and grow.

Check your expectations. You didn't lose strength or mobility overnight, and you're not going to instantly transform your body either. Expecting too much too soon only leads to frustration. Try not to be discouraged by what you can't accomplish or how far you have to go to reach your goals. Instead of obsessing over results, focus on consistency. While the improvements in mood and energy levels may happen quickly, the physical payoff will come in time.

Making excuses for not moving or exercising? Yes, I've heard them. Some of the most common ones follow. Find solutions instead.

"I hate exercising."

If sweating in a gym or pounding a treadmill isn't your idea of a great time, try to find an activity that you do enjoy–such as dancing–or pair physical activity with something more enjoyable. Take a walk at lunchtime through a park. Walk laps in an air-conditioned mall while window shopping. Walk, run, or bike with a friend, or listen to your favorite music while you move. Find an activity you enjoy and do it.

"I'm too busy."

Even the busiest of us can find free time in our day for activities that are important. It's your decision to make exercise a priority. And don't think you need a full hour for a good workout. Short 5-, 10-, or 15-minute bursts of activity can prove very effective. So, too, can squeezing all your exercise into a couple of sessions over the weekend. If you're too busy during the week, get up and get moving during the weekend when you have more time. Find a way–there is always a way if you make it a priority.

"I'm too tired."

It may sound counterintuitive, but physical activity is a powerful pick-me-up that actually reduces fatigue and boosts energy levels in the long run. With regular exercise, you'll feel much more energized, refreshed, and alert. Movement brings you energy.

"I'm too fat," "I'm too old," or "My health isn't good enough."

It's never too late to start building your strength and physical fitness even if you're an older adult or a self-confessed couch potato who has never exercised before. Very few health or weight problems rule exercise out of the question, so talk to your doctor about a safe routine. Start now—because you can.

"Exercise is too difficult and painful."

"No pain, no gain" is an outdated way of thinking about exercise. Exercise shouldn't hurt. And you don't have to push yourself until you're soaked in sweat or every muscle aches to get results. You can build your strength and fitness by walking, swimming, or even playing golf, gardening, or cleaning the house. Consult with your physician to learn to exercise safely.

"I'm not athletic."

Still have nightmares from gym class in school? You don't have to be sporty or coordinated to get fit. Focus on easy ways to boost your activity level like walking, swimming, or even working more around the house. Anything that gets you moving will work. Focus on what you can do, and do that.

What can you do? How can you make everyday activities work for you? If you're not the kind of person who embraces a structured exercise program, try to think about physical activity as a lifestyle choice rather than a task to check off your to-do list. Look at your daily routine and consider ways to sneak in activity here and there. Even very small activities can add up over the course of a day. Try these:

Make chores count. House and yard work can be quite a workout, especially when done at a brisk pace. Scrub, vacuum, sweep, dust, mow, and weed. They all count.

Look for ways to add extra steps. Take the stairs instead of the elevator or escalator. Park farther from a building entrance, rather than right out front. Get off your train or bus one stop early. The extra walking adds up.

Ditch the car whenever possible. Instead of driving everywhere, walk or bike when the distance is doable.

Move at work. Get up to talk to co-workers, rather than phoning or sending an email. Take a walk during your coffee and lunch breaks. Use the bathroom on another floor. Walk while you're talking on the phone.

Working from home? No problem. Get up at timed intervals such as every 30 minutes or every hour. Set an alarm to remind you. Use an app on your phone that monitors this. Walk to the farthest point in your home and back. Repeat if you can.

Get up during commercial breaks. Simply take a walk during breaks and every half hour. Sitting for a prolonged period of time compromises circulation and leads to joint stiffness.

Owning a pet can often lead to a more active lifestyle. Playing with and taking a dog for a walk, hike, or run are fun and rewarding ways to fit movement into your schedule. Studies have shown that dog owners are far more likely to meet their daily exercise requirements than nonowners.

Not only can movement help you lead a better, more active life now, it can add years to your life. And we're not just talking about quantity, since these years tend to be high on quality, too. According to the Harvard Health Letter, "A study in the Nov. 6, 2012, PLoS Medicine finds that overweight or obese people who engage in leisure-time physical activity can extend their lives by as much as four years, compared with similar-weight people who do no such activity." It adds that, "Being active and maintaining a healthy weight add an even bigger benefit, boosting longevity by more than seven years. (Harvard Health Letter, Exercise can add years to your life) The findings are similar to those of a study reported in the July 2012 Harvard Health Letter, which found that fitness and fatness independently affect your heart and have a greater impact when combined." (Harvard Health Letter, Exercise benefits the heart)

Personally, I don't need research to tell me this. My parents provided this lesson to me in such a way that one told me what not to do, the other told me what to do. My mother led a sedentary life. She didn't work outside the home, so she was with my brother and me a lot and took care of pretty much everything that needed to be done in the home. In addition to not moving much or exercising, she smoked cigarettes for many years and only quit when I went away to college. In every memory I have of her, she was overweight and sat a lot—often with a heating pad on her back due to pain. She was stiff when she walked, especially in the morning, and it didn't take much activity for her to be short of breath. She only lived until she was 72, passing of lung cancer from years of smoking (even though she quit some

20 years prior). Her life was cut short and her last years were compromised to put it nicely.

My father, on the other hand, lived until he was almost 92. He was active as long as I can remember, except for his last years with advancing dementia. Safe to say, though, he lived a very good life until the age of 85. He was active and he was athletic. As I mentioned earlier, he played sports including ice hockey and softball until his mid-60s. He was not overweight and did not smoke. He lived much longer than my mother and many of those years were quality years. The evidence is straightforward to me. The results speak for themselves.

There is no time like the present to assess where you are and make a choice as to where you want to go. You can control your destiny. You can make good lifestyle choices to change your life. That is a privilege. Please do not underestimate it. It is powerful and it is in your hands right now. Are you beating yourself up because of bad choices you made in the past? Accept the fact that they are in the past. What's done is done. But know this–they are not your future. Your future is up to you right now and it's staring you in the face. Make the most of it.

A friend of mine just made the decision to lead a healthier life and she is rocking it right now. What spurred it on? She saw a picture of herself on a Facebook memory that popped up on her phone, and she said, "It made me sick." She added, "Here I was not too long ago looking so fit, so trim, and so healthy. Oh, that pissed me off." She got real with herself and decided she wanted that person back, the person in that memory. She is now biking or walking every day and she boasts that she feels great and her energy level is through the roof. Well played, my friend. This can be you, too.

Chapter 2 What You Can Do

How's it going for you so far? Let's have a heart-to-heart talk about this. Because, quite honestly, if we don't do a little soul searching, there's a good chance the lessons learned here won't have much staying power. You've made it this far into the book, so it must mean something to you. This tells me you want more. You want a healthier life. You want to move more. You've got plans that you want to see realized. Amen to that. How bad do you want it? Are you willing to do what it takes?

You've heard the definition of insanity, right? It is the belief and expectation that if you continue doing what you're doing, you'll get a different result. It just doesn't work that way. If you want more, you must do more. Hope is not a strategy. It takes understanding where you are and then taking deliberate, meaningful action to get you to your goal. This chapter is about mindset and how the right one can lead you to a fulfilling active life.

My life changed dramatically when my father passed away six years ago. I was lost. I was his caregiver for the last 18 years of his life, which included a diagnosis of dementia. We lived together after my mother died unexpectedly. I wanted to take care of him as we had always been close. His dementia was in the very early stages then, barely perceptible. I had just graduated from physical therapy school, which I pursued after getting laid off at my job at an advertising agency and getting divorced. Life happens, doesn't it?

Watching my father go through his battle with dementia was hard. He was getting robbed of what could have been some very good years. He took it with an amazing grace, though, and I tried my best to match it. Some say the most challenging times of our lives can give us strength. They can give us hope. This is my story. During all these years of caregiving and all these years of challenge and grief, I had this one persistent thought in my head. Over and over again, it rose up. I didn't tell others about it then. I thought they would probably think I was crazy. Yet, it persisted. In time, I believed it. I believed it completely and with all my heart and soul. And even though I didn't know how I would pull it off, I somehow knew this was my destiny.

I knew, without a shadow of a doubt, that my next years would be the best of my life. I knew it when my father got sicker and deeper into the abyss of dementia. I knew it when he asked me the same question at least five times in a row. I knew it when I had to hire help to keep him safe. I knew it when I had to take his car keys away from him. I knew it when the police brought my father home in the middle of the night after he wandered off. I knew it when I placed him in a local assisted living facility with a memory care unit. These last two events nearly crushed me. Bless all the caregivers out there who are helping those we love to be healthy and safe.

I guess you could say I refused to be crushed. And because of all that I experienced, I promised myself I would live my life to the best of my ability and I would start as soon as possible. We just don't know how much time we have.

When my father passed away, my mission to care for him was complete. I wasn't perfect at the caregiving role, but I was able to keep him relatively healthy, safe, and as happy as possible. Goal achieved. He was worth every minute of it. I am not the same person who said I would take care of my father. I am much better.

In the six years since my father passed, I still believe that my best life is ahead of me. And here's the best part. I am living it now. I am helping adults make their next years their best years with meaningful movement. This is the reason I still practice as a physical therapist. This is the reason for my training business and my publishing and community education efforts. This is where it's at for me. I love every single minute of it. Truth be known, I have more dreams, too. I'll save that for another time. I am making my next years my best years.

You can, too. Embrace hope. Embrace what matters to you. Embrace living your dreams. With intent and meaning, anything is possible. Do it because you can.

Living your best life should include movement. It must include movement. After my father passed, I enrolled in personal development education, and some of the same strategies I learned there can help you improve your physical health. Movement is what this book is about, after all. Here, I will share with you some ways to improve your health, fitness, and quality of life. If they can work for me, they can work for you.

Five Steps to Meaningful Movement

Defy Aging

You are programmed. I am programmed. We all are programmed. From the day we were born, we have been programmed. It's time to press the reset program and download some new information.

Ageism is a buzz word these days. When I first heard it, I didn't understand what it meant. In the dictionary, it is described as, "prejudice or discrimination against a particular age-group and especially the elderly." (Merriam-Webster.com dictionary, ageism)

According to the World Health Organization:

> Ageism is the stereotyping, prejudice, and discrimination against people on the basis of their age. Ageism is widespread and an insidious practice which has harmful effects on the health of older adults. For older people, ageism is an everyday challenge. Overlooked for employment, restricted from social services and stereotyped in the media, ageism marginalizes and excludes older people in their communities.
>
> Ageism is everywhere, yet it is the most socially "normalized" of any prejudice, and is not widely countered—like racism or sexism. These attitudes lead to the marginalization of older people within our communities and have negative impacts on their health and well-being.
>
> (World Health Organization, Healthy Ageing)

As I learn more about ageism, it is not just discrimination. It is more insidious than that. It is the expectation that as we get older, we become weaker, we lose flexibility, and we lose our balance. It is the belief that we need more help and that we can't do it all ourselves. It is the belief, to some, that we can't live on our own. It is the belief we are in God's waiting room.

A client of mine, Jane, noticed her balance was getting worse. She was in her mid-60s and wondered if something else was going on in her body. She went to her family doctor who then referred her to an orthopedic physician. She met with this specialist with one thing in mind, and that was to find out what was wrong and to identify what she could do to improve her balance. He examined her, and when he was finished, he said to her, "Well, Jane, you are getting older." No. No. No. Shame on him. This is ageism, front and center. This is wrong to me on many fronts. First, was he indeed overlooking some other reason for the imbalance? Second, research shows that even though balance declines with age, you can help reverse these effects with exercise and training. You do not need to be afraid. You should be encouraged to take action and move.

It is unfair when others slap us with generalizations and discrimination. What is just as destructive, though, is when we do it to ourselves. Unfortunately, many of us have been programmed to accept compromised mobility as we age–just because we are older. We have to become more aware of the filters we use, both for ourselves and others. I am guilty of it, too, but I am intent on reprogramming myself to know better.

When I lived in New York, I created a publishing company for my books. Because of my passion for helping older adults, I named my new LLC Aging Well Now. I even packaged my community education into an initiative called the Aging Well Academy. I was proud of what I was doing– and I still am. But I learned something, thanks to one of my students. One day, a participant in one of my classes did me a favor and helped me realize something when she asked, "Why do you call it Aging Well Now? We know we are aging. So what? What we really want to do is live well now regardless of how old we are." She got it and I didn't. Thanks, friend, for setting me on a stronger path. She was able to describe my mission better than I was.

What is your self-talk? I was 52 years old and I wanted to start a new physical therapy practice. My first thought was, *Am I crazy? I'm too old to start something this big. What am I thinking?* True story. I was my biggest stumbling block. I was my biggest barrier. I reacted initially based on my beliefs and my previous programming. However, once I did a little research, I learned that the fastest growing segment of new business was being started by adults over 50. Wow. This was eye opening. I was helping to set trends. It's all in your perspective.

Challenge your beliefs; challenge your self-talk. Where is it coming from? What are the facts? Fact is, you might be capable of so much more than you think.

I hope that you'll realize all the choices you have and you'll choose to keep moving. I hope that by reading this book, you'll learn that you can improve your flexibility, strength, and balance at any age. That's right, any age. So what if you're 80. You can. You're 92? You can, too. You're 102? Yes, you can.

Take Daily Committed Action

It takes *daily committed action* to reach your goals. You can learn ways, many ways, to move and to keep moving. How you choose to move is up to you.

Let's break down this sentence:

Daily. Find a way, every day, to move. There is a lot to choose from. Walk the dog. Clean a room. Do some food prep for that special meal you want to cook this week. Get outside and work in the garden. Sweep out the garage or patio. Go to the gym or swim in a pool. Take a walk with a neighbor you haven't seen in a while. Schedule a golf game. Go for a bike ride. The opportunities are endless. Move daily.

Committed. Here's where goals and intent come into play. You don't have to decide right now your level of commitment, but it will come soon. You will understand what is at stake. Know this also. You are making a commitment even if you choose to stay where you are. If you decide not to change, you have still made a choice. I encourage you to learn the facts, trust those around you, and think long and hard about what matters to you. The smart choice for you will show itself.

Action. Hope is not a strategy. Make a habit out of living a healthy and fit life. I've heard it said that it takes 30 days of consistent action to make something a habit. A habit takes conscious thought out of the equation. You don't think about taking a walk. You just go do it. It is not up for discussion. It just happens.

Taking action means doing something. If you're a planner and like to schedule moving in your calendar, go for it. If you like building spreadsheets to create a plan for you to follow, do it. Just follow through on your planning. There is no time for analysis paralysis. Pick something and just start. I'll offer you ideas later in this book on how to get started all the way to what specifically you can do based on your current activity level. We all have our own starting point, and that's okay. As Nike, says, "Just do it."

Ask for Help

You don't have to do this alone. In fact, those who ask for help tend to reach higher levels of achievement than those who don't. You only know what you know. How can you possibly expect anything more? Others can show you new ways of moving, new ways of living your life.

Trusted sources include your physician, physical therapist, occupational therapist, professional trainer, or mentor. They all can be part of your movement and fitness team. When I turned to a professional coach after my father died, the universe provided me with the guidance I needed. I could not have reached the point I am at today without it. It's just that simple. I worked hard. I had to go down some roads I didn't want to travel– a journey that was necessary for me to see what was possible and to trust that all my work would pay off. And the returns just keep coming.

As a physical therapist, I learned a long time ago that I'm not just giving my patients an exercise to do. I am giving them the tools to get their life back. They can think of better things to do with their time. If they are with me, it's because they are hurting. Something happened and life is no longer the same. They want it back or they want it to be the best it can be. That's what I am there for. It's not just an exercise or movement I am providing. It is so much more.

One of my current virtual class participants recently told me, "This COVID-19 quarantine is doing a number on me. I am weaker and I have less energy. I'm hurting more, too. I'm not going out and I'm just not moving as much," said Karen. "I need your class. I need to get moving."

Ask for help, put in the work, and get back to those activities you enjoy.

Be with Like-Minded People

I have heard this many times from many people and I believe it to be true: You are the average of the five people with whom you spend the most time. Go ahead and crunch some numbers. If you have five numbers and you add them up and divide by five, you will always get the average of the five numbers. Always.

Now think of the five people with whom you spend the most time. Do they value moving, exercise, and activity as much as you do? Do they go out and walk or bike every morning? Are they active in their community? Do they have more energy than those who do not move much? Keep in mind that you are the average of those five people in ways such as your weight, your activity level, and likely even your wealth.

To improve your average, get to know those who move more than you. Spend time walking with them, talking with them, socializing with them. Who knows? You may lift up the others in your life who don't move as much now. Once they see what movement is doing for you, they are going to want some of that, too.

Maybe you enjoy walking so much with your neighbors and friends that you form a club. You really learn to enjoy each other, support each other, and cheer each other on in recognition of various achievements. You form a community of strong, like-minded people, and you change lives as a result– including your own. How cool is that? Be the one who inspires others.

Take Responsibility for Your Results

Own your results. Don't complain, blame others, or justify your situation. As I said before, just do it. Start moving and keep moving. Ask for help to provide accountability for your actions. Checking in with your new walking club every day is accountability. Having a buddy when going to the gym is accountability. Promising your spouse that you will ride your bike with him or her is accountability. These all help you take responsibility for your results. Accountability is great at helping you create habits. You may be at a point when you don't see the benefits yet, but you still made a commitment to move. Let accountability be that bridge between action and habit.

You are stronger than you think. I have been blessed to work with many wonderful patients and clients during my 25 years of practice. It has been a privilege to watch them learn what they can do. Years ago, I received a lovely card from one of my homecare patients, Barbara, soon after I discharged her. She had broken her hip during a fall and had it surgically repaired. She wrote, "You showed me I could get better and I did it faster than I ever thought possible. I didn't know what I could do. Thank you so much for giving me my life back."

Bob was a participant in my Buff Bones® Chair Class a few years ago. It was a joy to watch him as he cultivated an awareness that his body could do more than he thought. When asked to move his arms a certain way in class, he responded, "I didn't know I could move this much until you asked me. I can do this."

Others and I have the skills to help you move safely. Reach out and get the help you want and deserve. You just need the special skill to want to move and believe that you can.

Activity #1

I hope this chapter helped you come to a place where you want more. I highly recommend that you start a journal and use it to help identify a path for you to take once you finish this book. You may also use the Notes pages at the back of this book. There are a total of four activities, and each one will appear at the end of several chapters in this book. Please take the time to work through these. The plan you will create has its roots in medical strategic planning that I learned in physical therapy school.

For this activity, I want you to think about your status right now and reflect on the notion of creating a healthier and better life for yourself. Title this *Subjective*. Here are some questions to help you get started. How do you feel? Are you happy, content? If not, why? Do you want something more? If so, what do you want? How badly do you want it? What jazzes you? What is your self-talk? What do you want to be, do, or have?

Include everything that comes into your mind. Don't judge it. Accept it, write it down, and move on. Write everything down and return to it if something new pops into your head. Be honest. As you continue reading, add anything more that comes to mind. This is your starting point for the remaining activities in this book.

Good luck and have fun with it.

Chapter 3 What Really Happens When We Age

Our bodies are nothing short of a miracle. Waking up in the morning typically triggers the following routine. We move our limbs and our body to roll over and sit at the edge of the bed. We see what's around us. We stand and go to the bathroom. We wash our hands and brush our teeth. We shower and eat breakfast, and some of us go to work. We come home, eat dinner, spend time with our family, and then go to sleep. We take for granted all our body does to allow this to happen in a given day. So much happens behind the scenes to allow us to live to the best of our ability. It's truly amazing.

And that's just one day in, hopefully, your long life. But what happens over your lifespan? How does your body react to advancing age, which is what this book is about? You can be sure, you change. You can see it in the mirror, can't you? You can feel it, can't you? Our bodies change as we age. To study this further, let's identify the major systems of the human body.

Physiologically, there are 11 body systems that combine to keep your body healthy over your lifespan. Can you remember them all from health class in high school? Here they are with a brief description of their role:

Cardiovascular and Circulatory. Includes the heart, arteries, and veins to circulate blood throughout the body. Delivers oxygen and nutrients to organs and cells while carrying their waste products away. Also keeps the body's temperature in a safe range.

Digestive and excretory. Absorbs nutrients and removes waste.

Endocrine. Has hormones that influence the function of our body.

Integumentary and exocrine. Consists of skin, hair, nails, sweat, and exocrine glands.

Immune and lymphatic. Helps protect your body from foreign or harmful substances. Examples are bacteria, viruses, toxins, cancer cells, and blood or tissues from another person. The immune system makes cells and antibodies that destroy these harmful substances.

Muscular. Enables the body to move using muscles and also provides support to the body as well as heat.

Nervous. Collects information from the senses via nerves and the brain to tell our muscles to contract and thus cause physical actions.

Renal and urinary. Has kidneys that filter the blood to produce urine to get rid of waste.

Reproductive. Includes the organs required for the production of offspring.

Respiratory. Brings air into the lungs to absorb oxygen and remove carbon dioxide.

Skeletal. Has bones that maintain the structure of the body and its organs.

Various theories about aging are discussed in the literature. In reality, no one knows exactly how and why people change as they get older. Some theories are based in genetics. That is, that one or more genes in the cell nucleus dictate cellular energy. Another theory states that changes in our bodies come from damage. This could be the result of naturally occurring chemical reactions that begin to produce irreversible defects. Damage may also occur from wear and tear on the body or byproducts of metabolism. Yet a third theory points to a growing imbalance among various body systems. Here it is thought that the brain, endocrine system, and immune system gradually begin to malfunction and produce imbalance among various body systems.

It is important to note that no single process can explain all the changes. Aging is complex, and most gerontologists (people who study aging) believe it is the result of a lifelong series of changes and influences. These influences can range from heredity, environment, culture, diet, exercise, past illnesses, and likely other factors as well. Regardless of the theory, the fact is that every one of our systems changes with age. The rate of change and the extent of change are unique to each individual, according to the National Institutes of Health. (NIH, National Institute on Aging)

Some systems begin aging as early as age 30. Here is a brief overview of some of the changes we encounter as we age by system.

Cardiovascular and Circulatory Systems

The main artery from the heart (aorta) becomes thicker, stiffer, and less flexible. This makes blood pressure higher and makes the heart work harder, which may lead to thickening of the heart muscle (hypertrophy). The other arteries also thicken and stiffen. In general, most older people have a moderate increase in blood pressure.

Receptors called baroreceptors monitor the blood pressure and make changes to help maintain a fairly constant blood pressure when a person changes positions or is doing other activities. The baroreceptors become less sensitive with aging. This may explain why many older people have orthostatic hypotension, a condition in which the blood pressure falls when a person goes from lying or sitting to standing. This causes dizziness because less blood flows to the brain.

Normally, the heart continues to pump enough blood to supply all parts of the body. However, an older heart may not be able to pump blood as well when you make it work harder. This leads to decreased endurance, which means you have less tolerance to perform an activity over time.

Digestive and Excretory Systems

As you grow older, the body produces less stomach acid and less saliva, thereby slowing your digestion.

The muscles in the digestive tract become stiffer, weaker, and less efficient. Your tissues are also more likely to become damaged because new cells aren't forming as quickly as they once did.

Aging usually brings on more medications and these alone can affect your digestive tract negatively. These can include but are not limited to gastroesophageal reflux disease (GERD), peptic ulcers, heartburn, and constipation.

Endocrine System

Hormones are like the police of your body and control the target organs. Some organ systems have their own internal control systems along with or instead of hormones. As we age, changes naturally occur in the way body systems are controlled. Some target tissues become less sensitive to their controlling hormone. The quantity of hormones produced may also change.

The thyroid gland produces hormones that help control metabolism. Metabolism slows over time, beginning at about age 20.

In women, estrogen and prolactin levels often decrease significantly. Testosterone levels usually decrease gradually as men age. These changes can contribute to many things including decreased bone density. See more information about this in the Skeletal section.

Integumentary and Exocrine Systems

Skin changes are among the most visible signs of aging. Evidence of increasing age includes wrinkles and sagging skin. Whitening or graying of the hair is another obvious sign of aging.

With aging, the outer skin layer (epidermis) thins, even though the number of cell layers remains unchanged.

Changes in the connective tissue reduce the skin's strength and elasticity.

The sweat glands produce less sweat. This makes it harder to keep cool. Your risk for overheating or developing heatstroke increases.

Aging skin repairs itself more slowly than younger skin. Wound healing may be up to four times slower. This contributes to pressure ulcers and infections. Diabetes, blood vessel changes, lowered immunity, and other factors also affect healing.

Immune and Lymphatic Systems

The immune system becomes slower to respond. This increases your risk of getting sick. Flu shots or other vaccines may not work as well or protect you for as long as expected.

There are fewer immune cells in the body to bring about healing. This reduces the ability to resist infection.

The immune system's ability to detect and correct cell defects also declines. A type of cell called a T cell is responsible for circulating through the body to help detect infection and with aging, it circulates more slowly.

Muscular System

Lean body mass decreases. This decrease is partly caused by a loss of muscle tissue (a type of atrophy called sarcopenia). Muscle changes often begin in the 20s in men and in the 40s in women.

Loss of muscle results in loss of mobility, agility, and flexibility.

Muscles may become rigid with age, which makes them less responsive when we need them, for example to catch a fall. This change also limits the range of motion of joints, which can make movement painful and decrease our ability to move correctly.

Nervous System

Your brain and spinal cord lose nerve cells and weight. Neurogenesis, the creation of new nerve cells, decreases with age. Nerve cells may begin to pass messages more slowly than in the past as a result.

Slowing of thought, memory, and thinking is a normal part of aging. This is called normal cognitive decline. This is not dementia where mental decline impacts your everyday life. Dementia and severe memory loss are not a normal part of aging.

Renal and Urinary Systems

The bladder wall changes. The elastic tissue becomes tough and the bladder becomes less stretchy. The bladder cannot hold as much urine as before. The bladder muscles weaken. Aging increases the risk of bladder and other urinary tract infections (UTIs).

Reproductive System

Aging changes in the female reproductive system result mainly from changing hormone levels. One clear sign of aging occurs when menstrual periods stop permanently. This is known as menopause.

Aging changes in the male reproductive system may include changes in testicular tissue, sperm production, and erectile function. These changes usually occur gradually.

These changes are closely tied to changes in the urinary system for both men and women.

Respiratory System

Bones become thinner and change shape. This can change the shape of your ribcage. As a result, your ribcage cannot expand and contract as well during breathing.

The muscle that supports your breathing, the diaphragm, becomes weakened, which may prevent you from breathing enough air in or out.

These changes in your bones and muscles may lower the oxygen level in your body. Also, less carbon dioxide may be removed from your body. Symptoms such as tiredness and shortness of breath can result.

Aging also causes the air sacs to lose their shape and become less elastic. Therefore, they are not as efficient.

Older people are at increased risk for:

- Lung infections such as pneumonia and bronchitis

- Shortness of breath

- Low oxygen level

- Abnormal breathing patterns, resulting in problems such as sleep apnea (episodes of stopped breathing during sleep)

Skeletal System

People lose bone mass or density as they age, especially women after menopause. The bones lose calcium and other minerals. If there aren't enough reserves left in the bone, osteoporosis and osteopenia may occur. Adults with decreased bone density are more prone to fractures than adults with normal bone density.

The joints become stiffer and less flexible. Fluid in the joints may decrease. The cartilage may begin to rub together and wear away. Minerals may deposit in and around some joints (called calcification).

———

Stay with me here. I hope you can appreciate that no one system is independent of another. For example, hormone levels impact so many other systems. The reproductive system changes are often tied to urinary symptoms such as an enlarged prostate for men. The body is amazing and so complex, which explains how individuals differ in how they age.

Now you're probably thinking, "Well gee, Nancy. Thanks for this pep talk." I share this information with you because I need to arm you with the facts. Information is powerful if we use it the right way. Information is powerful if we use it the right way. That's not a typo–that sentence is worth repeating. We need to use it. Remember when we discussed mindset and the importance of approaching each challenge with, "How can I?" This is up to us, no one else. Not your husband or wife, not your brother or sister, not your friends or your neighbors. It rests with you. And thank goodness. Because that puts us square in the driver's seat as to what we do for us. That thinking, my friends, is powerful. We got this, which leads me to the next chapter. It's time for the good news. Here, you will better understand the miracle of movement and appreciate what it can do to help reverse what our bodies are doing as we move through this life.

.

Chapter 4 Why Movement Is Good for Us

Let's review where we are. We learned that every one of our systems changes with age. I have gone on to say that movement and exercise can help reverse the changes in our bodies due to aging. Movement is your fountain of youth. Now, I show you how.

Cardiovascular and Circulatory Systems

Regular exercise makes your heart stronger and its ability to pump blood increases. This is why elite athletes have a low resting heart rate compared to the average person.

Exercise stimulates your circulatory system and enhances the removal of toxins from blood. It also increases the flow of oxygenated blood in the body.

Exercise makes your arteries more flexible. This improves circulation and helps lower your blood pressure. This also helps your body deal with sudden elevation of blood pressure due to intense physical activity.

Exercise reduces inflammation in the body. Regular exercise reduces C-reactive protein (CRP) whose presence indicates inflammation in the body. Inflammation is currently being studied extensively as it is implicated in many chronic diseases including coronary heart disease, diabetes, and even dementia.

Exercise burns calories and is critical for weight control. Hypertension and diabetes are the most common diseases found in overweight people.

Digestive and Excretory Systems

Exercise improves blood flow throughout the body. Keep your body moving with regular exercise, and you can keep your digestive tract moving, too. Consistent exercise can also help you avoid constipation, gas, and bloating

Endocrine System

Exercise boosts the number of hormones circulating in your body and strengthens receptor sites on target organ cells. Your endocrine response to exercise can improve organ function, physical appearance, and state of mind. Exercise improves insulin sensitivity and reduces the reliance on insulin injections.

Thus, exercise can reduce your reliance on medications to control diabetes.

Integumentary and Exocrine Systems

Regular exercise improves circulation and thus promotes healthy skin. Because exercise increases circulation, it helps wounds heal faster.

Immune System

Movement and exercise help improve the circulation of your immune cells. As a result, these immune cells can roam the body more quickly and more effectively to find pathogens and eradicate them.

Exercise consistently and you have a powerful housekeeping activity that helps your immune system patrol the body and detect and then rid the body of bacteria and viruses.

———

This has never been more important than in the year 2020. Life appeared out of control, and movement let us reclaim some of it back. Allow me to expand on this a bit more here.

As I write this, our country–in fact our entire world–is grappling with the pandemic known as COVID-19, the novel coronavirus disease. COVID-19 is a respiratory illness that was first identified in Wuhan, Hubei, China, in December 2019. According to the CDC, reported illnesses have ranged from mild symptoms to severe illness and death. Symptoms appear 2 to 14 days after exposure, said the CDC, with the most common being fever, cough, and shortness of breath. Older adults and people who have severe underlying medical conditions like heart or lung disease or diabetes seem to be at higher risk for developing more serious complications from COVID-19 illness. The virus is thought to spread mainly from person to person in close contact, through respiratory droplets produced when an infected person coughs or sneezes. (CDC, Coronavirus Disease 2019)

Social distancing is now a thing. Isolation, quarantines, and major city and state lockdowns have occurred as a result of this highly contagious and dangerous disease. Financial markets suffered initially as a result of this pandemic, and unemployment continues, as of this writing, at a very high rate. It is safe to say that all are affected in one way or another. And, they have been affected in ways never before seen.

I must admit that when I first heard older people were at much greater risk for complications if infected with the novel COVID-19, I was scared. I wondered, *What is old age? Is it 65 and older? At what age are we older?* In regard to this disease, we are still learning the demographics. Regardless, what is it about this older generation–arguably more health conscious than previous generations–that would make us more vulnerable to complications from this virus (or any virus really) than younger folks? You learned it earlier, and it can be answered with this one word–age. That's it, age.

As you get older, your immune system does not usually respond as quickly or as forcefully to pathogens as it did when you were younger. With movement, however, you can improve that. According to Mark Moyad, M.D., M.P.H., Jenkins/Pokempner Director of Preventive and Alternative Medicine at the University of Michigan Medical Center, activity causes your body's antibodies and white blood cells to circulate more rapidly, which means they may be able to detect and zero in on bugs more quickly. Being active also lowers stress hormones, which reduces your chances of getting sick, Moyad adds. (Hallie Levine, AARP)

According to Hallie Levine, research suggests that exercise's effects may be directly relevant to virus fighting. According to a recent study published in the British Journal of Sports Medicine, of 1,002 people surveyed, those who exercised at least five days a week had almost half the risk of coming down with a cold as those who were more sedentary. If they did get one, they reported less severe symptoms. (Hallie Levine, AARP)

Susan M. Friedman, MD, MPH Professor of Medicine, URMC, says "Exercise daily, aiming for at least 30 minutes of moderate activity per day. Make sure that you work up a sweat. This virus has the highest impact on people's hearts and lungs, so you want to make sure that they are in as good a shape as possible if you get the virus." (Friedman, Susan M., MD, MPH, A Lifestyle Medicine Approach to COVID-19)

Six Ways to Boost Your Immune System

Now, more than ever, folks understand the value of keeping our immune systems at the top of their game. Besides exercise, here are six other ways you can boost your immune system.

- Eat more of a plant-based diet, and remove processed food from your diet.

- Avoid smoking or inhaling any substance that can be toxic to the lungs.

- Get enough sleep that is restful and restorative.

- Connect with family and friends, and cultivate healthy relationships.

- Spend time outside. Go for a morning walk, and enjoy fresh air when you can.

- Manage stress. Movement and all of the above can help with stress. Seek professional help if it is too difficult to tackle alone.

Muscular System

Your muscles need blood and oxygen to remove cellular waste and produce energy for physical activity. Exercise provides this.

- Exercise can improve your endurance, which is required for physical activity over time.

- Exercise improves your strength, allowing you to participate more effectively in any activity from your normal daily routine to vigorous sports.

- Exercise improves coordination and balance allowing you to learn and master complex movement patterns.

Nervous System

Physical exercise promotes blood flow to your brain and helps reduce loss of brain cells.

Exercise helps improve communication between your nerves and muscles, which maximizes strength and function.

Renal and Urinary Systems

Regular exercise is considered a simple and natural way to improve kidney function.

Exercise helps keep you fit and healthy and can help you keep your weight in check. If you are overweight, it can lead to high blood pressure, which can put a lot of strain on the kidneys.

Reproductive System

The subtle physiological changes that come from exercise can benefit your odds of conceiving and boost fertility.

Exercise improves metabolism and circulation, both of which contribute to better egg production.

Regular activity also optimizes your reproductive system by stimulating the endocrine glands, which secrete hormones that help eggs grow.

Respiratory System

Physical exercise improves lung function and efficiency.

Exercise helps facilitate transport of oxygen to all the cells in the body.

Lying in bed or sitting for long periods can allow mucus to collect in the lungs. This puts you at risk of lung infections. Movement and exercise decrease your risk of infection.

Skeletal System

Exercise, especially weight-bearing exercise and resistance training, can help improve bone density and decrease the risk of osteoporosis and osteopenia.

With exercise, you can build strong bones at any age.

Exercise improves joint mobility and increases synovial fluid circulation in joints. This leads to improved joint health and helps reduce the symptoms of degenerative conditions including osteoarthritis.

––––––––––

Have you noticed that movement and exercise improve the function of every system in our body? Our bodies are remarkable. Perhaps you've identified with some of the conditions noted here in this chapter. If you have, be sure to keep reading to dive into some of the most common chronic conditions we experience as we age. And, you guessed it, movement plays a critical role in managing each one.

It's important that you know the facts about movement. Physiologically, it performs quite a miracle. Our bodies are amazing. Movement is just as amazing. Let's see what else movement can do for us.

Chapter 5 Movement's Gifts

Movement and exercise can help improve your mobility and health in each and every area we just discussed. Even with the normal physiological changes your body goes through as you age, you can help reverse these changes with movement and exercise. There is no greater gift.

Always remember the freedom you have in how you choose to move. Even more, you can choose to move and benefit from it at any age. Every day of your life you can become stronger and more fit, improve your balance, and enjoy your life more. Every day. Age is no longer an excuse. This stops now.

Let me share some other of movement's gifts. Here you will learn how movement and exercise change your body and how they can make you feel. These, too, are the result of physiological changes that we learned about in the previous chapter. The focus or perspective is just a little different. Here is what movement can do for you:

Decrease Pain

Exercise prompts the body to produce endorphins that interact with opiate receptors in the brain to reduce our perception of pain. Endorphins act similarly to drugs such as morphine and codeine but without the addiction.

Painful joints are often due to muscle tightness, which alters normal forces in a joint. For example, knee pain can be due in part to tight hamstring muscles at the back of the thigh and tight quadriceps muscles at the front of the thigh. This phenomenon can apply to all joints.

Stretching alone can eliminate pain. I use it all the time. You may recall I have a condition called spondylolisthesis, a structural deformity at my lumbar spine. I know when I'm getting tighter than normal by the pain I feel in my low back. If I can catch it soon enough, I can go through my stretching routine and abolish the pain in about 15 minutes. And it stays away. That may be why I think of stretching as dessert. It is a most satisfying treat. I love to stretch. I also think of it as an investment in my next activity whether it be just working out or playing sports. It helps to set me up for success. I highly recommend it.

Decrease Stiffness

Movement and exercise can decrease stiffness. Consider degenerative osteoarthritis (OA), for example. OA often manifests itself with painful and stiff joints. Let's take the knee again as an example. If you perform continuous, low resistance movement at your knee such as riding a stationary bicycle and perform it even 10 minutes, you will likely decrease stiffness in that joint. One reason is synovial fluid. Deep in the joint is a capsule, and inside that capsule is this synovial fluid that coats the bony surfaces of that joint. This fluid has oxygen and nutrients that feed your joints, too. As a result, friction is reduced and the joint moves more freely.

Increase Range of Motion

Exercise that pushes the limits of movement in a restricted joint due to soft tissue tightness (absent of some other kind of blockage) can improve the range of motion of that joint. Physical therapists and other movement therapists measure joint movement in degrees and are skilled at knowing when motion is normal or limited.

Increase Strength and Power

Movement and exercise can increase muscle strength and power if they are designed to do so. Muscles are the structures that produce force and when properly loaded with resistance, they can become stronger over time.

Muscles move our bodies. Strength is critical as we age as it allows us to do the activities we want to do and gives us strong legs to maximize our balance.

Opening a jar, opening a door, climbing a step, rolling in bed—all of these require strength to perform them effectively.

Improve Balance

Activities and exercises that challenge our balance will help improve it.

Balance is achieved and maintained by a complex set of sensorimotor control systems that include sensory input from vision (sight), proprioception (touch), and the vestibular system (motion, equilibrium, and spatial orientation). As therapists, we are trained to isolate systems and train them to work more efficiently.

Safe mobility relies on good balance. It is key to aging independently.

Improve Mobility

Mobility here is defined as walking, but it also includes moving from one surface to another. The latter includes sit-to-stand activities and can even include getting in and out of a car.

Movement and exercise can improve your mobility. Compromised mobility is one of the most common reasons people are referred to a physical therapist.

Improve Ability to Perform Activities of Daily Living (ADL)

Specialized movement and exercise can improve your ability to perform activities of daily living. These activities include dressing, bathing, and kitchen tasks among others. Occupational therapists specialize in this area and are a wonderful resource for you to consider if necessary.

Improve Endurance

Endurance is your ability to perform an activity or task over time. Walking is an endurance activity. So is biking. Decreased endurance frequently exhibits itself as shortness of breath or undue fatigue.

Movement and exercise can improve your endurance, especially those activities that are considered aerobic in nature. That is, you use oxygen continuously throughout the activity. This can be trained with appropriate exercise.

———

Movement and exercise can also provide these great benefits:

- Improve your mood

- Improve your sleep

- Improve your energy

- Decrease stress

- Decrease risk of depression

Endorphins, which help reduce pain, also play a major role in the above benefits. In fact, some medical professionals prescribe regular exercise as a treatment for mild to moderate depression and anxiety. Meditation and yoga are known for their stress-relieving and relaxing effects, which may be partially due to an endorphin release. Managing stress is important to reduce cortisol levels and optimize your immune system.

You may recall I am writing much of this book during the COVID-19 pandemic. Now, more than ever, it is important to stay positive, active, and connected in an effort to reduce stress and the risk of depression. There are some creative people out there doing what they can to feel better now. I just love what they are doing. See if their ideas are activities you might want to try, or maybe they will give you an idea to do something you like even more.

Twenty Rides in 2020

Karen loves to go camping with her family, and they do so frequently throughout the summer. She, her husband, and their young son have made a commitment to do 20 bike rides in 2020. Not only do they enjoy the rides together, but they have a lot of fun planning them, too. They are learning and exploring while they take good care of themselves and each other. Bravo.

Local Hikes with Friends

Mary enjoys hiking and exploring various parks where she lives. She started posting pictures of her surroundings on social media. Then, she invited others to join her. They pick a place and time. They meet there and hike the area together (while social distancing). They take their cameras, too, and now others, including me, can see more pictures from their adventures. I feel like I am with them. Thanks, friends, and cheers to staying connected in a healthy way.

Morning Walks

Susan takes a walk early every morning. She and her husband wander around and take pictures of interesting things and beautiful landscapes. These include anything from beautiful flowers to animal carvings out of wood. She provides a slice of life by posting her photos on social media, and I really enjoy seeing them. I know others do, too. Thanks for sharing the beauty that is all around us.

Sure, the pandemic is an extreme example of a challenging time to get out there and move. Other challenges come and go though, don't they? How can you stay active and connected? Maybe you like to hike. Make a pledge to hike 21 trails in 2021. Invite family and friends. What appeals to you and how can you inspire others to do the same? Make your pledge meaningful, and inspire others along the way. You will go a long way toward living a healthier life both physically and mentally.

In the following chapters, we are sharpening our focus as it pertains to movement. Movement can be any activity we do, right? Exercise is a form of movement–that is, it is an example of a type of movement. Furthermore, when we exercise, we can do it for fun and/or we can exercise for some specific purpose. That purpose might be to help recover from an injury. The purpose of exercise can also be born out of a desire to improve some aspect of your physical abilities. It then becomes purposeful and meaningful because you are trying to improve some specific activity. This activity might be walking or climbing the flight of stairs in your home. Maybe you want to be able to pick up your grandchildren with less back pain. Maybe you want to be able to walk longer with less shortness of breath. For some, exercise can be recreational in nature or sport specific. Examples of this include wanting to hit a golf ball farther or wanting to hit the tennis ball with more power. There are a million reasons (and likely more) you may want to improve your physical fitness so that you can participate in activities you enjoy.

There is a concept about more targeted exercise that we call prescriptive exercise, because the exercise is designed specifically for you with a goal in mind. The foundation of physical therapy, as well as other rehabilitation specialties such as occupational and speech therapy, is prescriptive exercise. As therapists, we are trained to think strategically and create a plan of care, for you and just for you, to help you reach your goals. That plan of care is largely prescriptive exercise. As you age, chances are you manage conditions that cannot be otherwise cured. Here enter prescriptive exercise where the benefits are ideal for you, the active adult, because they are designed for you and only you.

Activity #2

It's time to build on what you started in your journal. You have learned more about what movement can do for you. Please continue writing in your journal and title this section *Objective*. Try to identify the role movement has in your life right now and where you see opportunities how it can help you in the future. Answer the following questions: Where are you now in your movement journey? What are your strengths? What are your weaknesses? What do you like to do? What do you avoid? What are you good at? What are you not so good at? What is happening positively in your life right now that can help springboard you to new heights in the future?

Again, please be honest. Don't judge your thoughts. Just write them down as they come. As before, please feel free to add to this as more thoughts surface while you read the next chapters.

Keep up the great work. You are halfway there to an actionable plan for yourself. Congratulations.

Chapter 6 The Perfect Match

Prescriptive exercise is the result of a thorough assessment of your capabilities, resulting in a plan of care customized for you and targeted to meet your goals. That is what I do. That is what a physical therapist does. Moreover, I am a movement specialist. My career and lifelong passion has been devoted to movement, purposeful movement. Every day of my life, I am educating and, hopefully, inspiring an adult to move. I love what I do.

You may recall I first discovered physical therapy (PT) after my own injury in college. When hockey and sports were taken away from me, movement in the form of physical therapy brought them back. It often wasn't easy. Nothing worthwhile is. And it frequently hurt. But it was worth it. All of it was worth it. Movement continues to provide me health and happiness. Both personally and, yes, as a career. PT taught me how to move the right way. PT helped me feel better and live an active life. And PT, as it turns out, gave me so much more.

As a physical therapist, I help you move. What an honor. I really mean that. Sure, I've heard the jokes over the years. "PT means physical terrorist, right?" or "PT = Pain and torture." But you still came back for your next session. Thank you for that. You have allowed me to teach you and help heal you. You've allowed me to touch you and work out your overworked muscles or stretch your body to regain mobility. You've allowed me to move your body in a way that is healthy, not compromised. You've allowed me to apply modalities to your body in the form of heat, ice, electric stimulation, and anti-inflammatories to help you feel better and have less pain. I take that very seriously, and I'm privileged to have helped thousands upon thousands of you during my career. I will continue to help you as long as I can. I have touched a lot of people, but, more importantly, I've touched a lot of lives.

Maybe you're wondering what PT is and what the term rehabilitation (or rehab, for short) is all about. Let's first consider the definition of physical therapy.

Definition of physical therapy (also called physiotherapy)

> Therapy for the preservation, enhancement, or restoration of movement and physical function impaired or threatened by disease, injury, or disability that utilizes therapeutic exercise, physical modalities (such as massage and electrotherapy), assistive devices, and patient education and training.

Definition of rehabilitation

> Restoration especially by therapeutic means to an improved condition of physical function.

(Merriam-Webster.com dictionary)

So what is so special about the medical rehabilitation approach, and why do I call it the perfect match? There are some common approaches to PT and rehab that are ideal for the aging adult. Adults often manage chronic conditions, and physical therapists have specific training and experience in how to care for these conditions. That is why.

I'll let you in on a secret. It's called the SOAP note. No, it's not a very clean piece of paper. It is an acronym to describe how we think as clinicians and how we create a plan of care. It is how we document what we do in a structured, strategic, and goal-driven way. It has meaning, and you are at the center of its meaning. It's all about you. In fact, the action plan you are creating with the activities in this book is based specifically on this. Let me share it with you in the context of a medical professional such as a physical therapist evaluating a patient.

S = Subjective

This is a summary of your explanation as to why you have come seeking help. If you have pain, we ask more about that. We want to know how intense it is, where it is, and what it feels like (sharp, dull, throbbing, etc.). If a specific injury caused your symptoms, we want to know about that, too. We want to know how your life is compromised. We want to learn what it is that you can no longer do as a result. Our goal as rehab specialists is to try to get you back to your previous level of function.

O = Objective

This information comes from our physical examination. It includes anything relevant to your condition, which may include your ability to walk, your balance, your flexibility or range of motion, your strength, and any other pertinent information to help identify structures impacted.

A = Assessment

We then consider the subjective and objective information and create a clinical assessment of your condition. We include the physician's diagnosis if there is one and create a plan of care. We provide a prognosis for you and confirm (when appropriate) that physical therapy and rehab should help you recover and reach your goals. Both you and me, as the therapist, create short-term and long-term goals so we have something to work toward and can measure your progress while receiving care. These are critical when we reassess you later to determine if the plan of care is still appropriate.

P = Plan

This describes how we will implement the plan of care for you, including what therapeutic techniques will be used. Examples include stretching, strengthening, gait training, balance training, and modalities if needed. The plan will also include your recommended frequency of visits and the duration that the episode of care is expected to take (for example, 4 weeks, 6 weeks, 2 months, etc.).

———

A SOAP note leads to a purposeful and meaningful roadmap of activities to help you feel better, move better, and live better. If you are interested in knowing what PT can possibly do for you at this point, please consult with your physician to discuss your options. The best plan comes from a collaborative approach with your physician and other allied health professionals.

Like a roadmap, a SOAP note defines your starting point and gives you a target to work toward. I reveal it here because this map can also help you define your path to a more active life. I want you to know about and use this tool because it gives you the power to take action now. By reading and participating in the activities in this book, you are following this type of plan and are creating a meaningful and well-thought-out path to wellness that will improve your life. And it starts right now.

The rehab model of a SOAP note leads you forward to another place, a new place. If appropriate for you, it gives you hope. Your plan doesn't have to be in this form, but I highly recommend it be structured to provide a strategy to get you to your goal, regardless of your starting point.

Goal setting is at the heart of this. Think about this. What do you want? What do you want to do? What do you want to do again? Do you want to return to activities you enjoy? Do you want to have fun? Do you want to spend more time with your family and friends? C'mon. What do you want?

Physical therapy healed me and gave sports and hockey back to me. It gave me a future that I cherished then and still do. This thought process is what I rely on for myself to help me go even further. I am so not done yet. I may be knocking on the door of 60 years old, but I still want my next years to be my best years. To that end, I walk and bike regularly. I recently learned how to play pickleball. I golf at least once a week, sometimes twice. A few months ago, I shot an 80 for 18 holes—my best ever. I'm reinventing myself, and I'm so grateful for the opportunity to even just try. Your future is yours to design.

I didn't always have this mindset of strength and possibilities that lie before me. Some special people helped me understand it. One was Dr. Dale Fish who, at the time, was Dean of the PT program at SUNY University at Buffalo. Before even applying to the physical therapy program there, I made an appointment to visit with him and learn more about it. In some respects, I thought meeting with him was a little too early in the process as I hadn't even applied yet. I still had to complete two years of schooling to complete the prerequisite courses. Above and beyond that, I also had to score very high grades in these courses to be considered for this very competitive program.

Still, he met with me and was extremely gracious with his time and knowledge. I will never forget the mighty message he had for me. Instead of pointing out the obstacles in my path, he took a different approach. "Everything is in front of you," Dr. Fish said. "It's yours to make happen.

It's not like others who have already done the work (took the prerequisite courses). You can control your desired outcome here." Wow. Just wow. So much power was given to me by this man I had just met. He didn't know me from Adam then, but that didn't stop him from changing my life.

Sometimes we can't see our potential until someone else offers it to us. You are in the same space as I was. Here is my message to you. Everything in front of you is yours to create. It's yours to make happen. Do you want a better life? Do you want to spend more time with your family, your kids, and your grandchildren? Do you want to go out with your friends when they ask? Do you? You can.

How badly do you want it? For years, I have been teaching specialized fitness classes that help adults build strong bones. The class includes resistance training, core strengthening, fall prevention, and balance training. Participants know in advance that when enrolling in my mat class, they need to be able to get up and down from the floor. I remember one of my past participants vividly. She came to the first class using a cane and had a noticeable limp. I asked her if she could get up from the floor and she immediately said yes. However, when it came time to do it (and with a room full of 15 other participants watching her), it wasn't so easy. I offered to help her and she declined. Others also wanted to help but could only watch her struggle to do it. After a few attempts, she looked me in the eye and said sincerely, "I know I can do this." There was something about her that made me believe she could, and I think everyone in the room believed her, too. Very soon after, she did it. Without any help from anyone, she did it. The whole room applauded her.

She wanted it badly. So badly that she showed up every week and worked hard each and every class. She even practiced some of the exercises at home. After about a month (at once a week), she rose from her mat with greater ease and blended right in with the abilities of the others. She confessed later that when she started class, she wasn't going out much because her mobility was so limited. By the time classes ended for that 10-week session, she was out meeting friends for lunch every week. Determination will take you far, my friends. Everything in front of you is yours to create.

This rehab approach that I discuss in this chapter is universally beneficial. It does not discriminate. The rehab approach works for young people. It works for elite athletes. It works for weekend warriors. It also works for older adults who want to improve their fitness, their health, and their quality of life. It especially works for older adults like you, because chances are, you are managing chronic conditions that require ongoing management.

This leads me to another reason why the physical therapy and rehab model works so well for adults. Not only is it customized to your needs, it is likely more conservative than what you would find for the general population in your community. Because of the education required to become a physical therapist, you are more likely to start training at a safer place that is more appropriate and effective for you. As I mentioned earlier, please consult with your physician to help you find your best place to start.

Physical Therapy Versus Occupational Therapy—What's the Difference?

I'm often asked, What's the difference between a physical therapist (PT) and an occupational therapist (OT)?" Both are licensed professionals who graduated from an accredited program. There are exceptions, but generally a PT will work with someone with a condition below the waist. An OT works with those for ailments above the waist. Again, this is very general and often is dictated by the facility at which the therapists work. Both OTs and PTs can treat shoulder pain. Both OTs and PTs can be hand specialists. It's not black and white and as I said, please consult your local facility to see how to best proceed for your specific condition. It is widely accepted, though, that for ambulation (walking), mobility (getting from point A to point B), and balance issues, PT is the way to go. Again, legs are below the waist, so that guideline works consistently facility to facility.

––––––––

Not all movement specialists have the experience or interest, quite frankly, to work with adults over 50. Perhaps they specialize in pediatric care, for example. Look for the professionals who know how to manage chronic disease. Rehab specialists such as physical and occupational therapists, know this. It is part of our training. It is often a part of our experience.

A Different Perspective

Everyone's situation, needs, and desires are different. Not everyone can pull off what my class participant did with her mobility. I offer another way to think about this. At the very least, maintain your current health and ability to move. From this point forward, don't lose what you have today. Make sure tomorrow you can do what you can do today. This can apply to many things in our life, but here, it applies to movement. It includes getting from your bed to your bathroom in the morning. It includes changing your clothes, preparing breakfast, and sitting down to enjoy it. It includes going out to lunch with friends. It includes driving. You get the picture. The key is to keep moving as you do today.

Some of you may not want to move. My response is do it anyway. Don't sacrifice your life and your goals for what you want now. Move so you can have what you want most–and this includes your future and your goals. Please consider the examples of this chapter as you continue your personal action plan with the activities of this book. Use the SOAP note model to help define your next years. Revisit it often and add to it as your needs and desires change. This tool can work for you now and in the future. A good plan will grow with you. Don't just listen to me. Listen to my patients.

For the first 24 years of my physical therapy career, I lived in a small town in Upstate New York. I would often run into former patients at the local stores. I shopped at Wegmans routinely, which I miss dearly by the way. I know, it's a supermarket, but if you ever get the chance to go to a Wegmans, do it. You won't be disappointed. You'll understand why tourists go to Wegmans when they visit the area. It's an experience. But I digress.

I saw many of my patients in Wegmans. My record for seeing former patients at this local supermarket in one shopping trip is nine patients. That day, there were four in produce alone. "Thanks, Nancy, for giving me my arm back," one said as she raised her right arm overhead to show me her prized mobility. "Thanks, Nancy, for getting rid of my heel pain," said another. "I'm shopping again," said another while showing me her full cart. "Thanks, Nancy, because I don't need my walker or my cane anymore," said a patient who had suffered a stroke before I worked with him.

Another, a more formal gentleman, sent me a typed progress report every few months after his discharge. Occasionally, he would hand deliver it to me in the clinic so he could tell me in person how he was doing. He actually took time out of his life to prepare these notes and even hand deliver them to me.

These folks are proud of their accomplishments. So proud that they couldn't wait to tell me. They should be proud. They worked hard to recover and reclaim their life. I am proud of their will to succeed. I am here to tell you, from them, that it was worth it. All the hard work, the discomfort, the sweat, and very likely the tears. It was worth it to get their life back and to participate in the activities they enjoy.

Your body is the means to your dreams. I hope you can see that now. Movement can be your exercise. And exercise can be your movement. Exercise can be prescriptive in nature. You choose. If it challenges you in a doable, reasonable, and meaningful way, then do it. Treat your body with the respect it deserves. Nurture it. Make it the best it can be. Then watch your dreams come true.

Chapter 7 Miracle Drug for Chronic Conditions

Last October my husband and I moved into an over-55 community in central Florida. We love it here. There are over 800 residences ranging from villas to single family homes. Most are one story and we have access to a fitness center, three pools, tennis and pickleball courts, and more. It is a vibrant community with many active adults just like us. It is also a community filled with folks doing their best to manage chronic conditions. You can't reach 55 without going through some stuff, right?

Last week my husband and I left to do some grocery shopping when we saw our neighbor, Larry, out for a walk. We stopped and rolled down the window to say hello. Larry and Ellen live just down the street and we became fast friends just a few months ago.

"How's it going, Larry? Good to see you," I said.

"Oh, it's going," he said.

Larry has had his share of physical challenges and is now dealing with a flare-up. He is experiencing low back and hip pain and has seen physicians to help control it. He is currently enrolled in physical therapy and is diligent with his home exercise program.

"I just had another shot in my hip," he said. "I think it's helping." He recently had injections to his low back, too, and had a nerve ablation done. A nerve ablation is when nerve endings are cauterized to stop the signal of pain to an area. Larry is doing all he can to feel better and return to activities he enjoys. He belongs to the community golf league but hasn't played recently due to his pain. Also, he and his wife just postponed a trip to see their daughters up North, in part, due to Larry's current physical condition. I know this had to be hard on him, but Larry is still Larry and he is still smiling. He has a wonderful sense of humor.

"They tricked us," he said. "They really did. Who said these years are golden?"

I wish I had a dollar for all the times I've heard that from my patients. "These golden years aren't so golden," they would say. Still, so many soldier on and do whatever it takes to feel better and stay active. Applause, applause.

When I first met Larry, his walk was memorable as his upper body would lurch side to side excessively with each step. He was pretty steady, but the compensations he showed were remarkable. Turns out, this was normal for him. When his recent flare-up occurred, he began to walk with a straight, single-point cane. He was not steady then and he certainly needed something more to support him. Today, Larry was walking with a four-wheeled walker with a seat. That is a lot of support and I was part shocked and part relieved to see him using it. With the walker, he could walk longer and more easily negotiate sidewalks and uneven ground. He could walk for exercise. And he improved his safety by reducing his risk for falls.

"I feel better when I move," said Larry. "So I move." More applause.

How many of you can relate to Larry and his situation right now? We all have our challenges, don't we? We have physical ailments that need attention, and typically they bring along emotional challenges, too. Larry's movement paid off. As I edit this chapter, Larry has since returned to playing golf, and he and Ellen rescheduled their trip to see their daughters and leave next week.

Put your faith in movement. We are not built to sit. We are built to move. What's more, what can help us live an active and healthy life when we are young can help us overcome limitations when we are older.

As this chapter continues, I will address five of the more common chronic conditions affecting older adults that do not have a cure. There is no magic pill either. In some severe cases, surgical intervention can help. An example of this might be a total knee replacement for a joint deteriorated by osteoarthritis. In my years of practice, though, I have learned that this rarely comes on suddenly. Surgery is often not the answer especially in the early stages of degenerative changes. This is when you manage it.

The five conditions I address here affect millions of people in this country alone. Space limits my ability to address all chronic conditions, but know the following ones are extremely common and their impact on you can be significant. They require awareness of your health and knowledge of the tools to help keep these conditions from worsening or causing other problems down the road. One common tool helps manage them all, and that is movement. They all require some form of movement to maintain or even improve their impact on you. I will describe the condition, share its impact on your health, and finally show you how movement can improve each one.

Osteoarthritis

What Is It?

Did you know there are over 100 types of arthritis conditions out there? The one we're discussing here is the most common and called osteoarthritis (OA). In general, it is an inflammation (any time you see a word ending with *itis*, it means inflammation) or swelling of one or more joints and, most commonly, occurs in the hands, hips, and knees. It is caused by damage or breakdown of joint cartilage between bones and is, therefore, considered degenerative.

According to the Centers for Disease Control and Prevention, osteoarthritis is defined as a wearing down of cartilage within a joint and the underlying bone begins to change. (CDC, Arthritis)

I liken OA to a road. Pretend the road you're driving on is the bone surface at a joint. A new road is smooth and flat and the ride is not bumpy. When you have OA, the road is full of cracks and maybe even some pot holes. The ride (or movement of the joint) is no longer smooth but is bumpy and often painful. Inflammation occurs as a result and over time, the road continues to worsen. This is consistent with OA as symptoms usually develop slowly and worsen over time.

Characteristics

OA causes pain, stiffness, decreased flexibility, and swelling in affected joints. Over time, mobility suffers and the joint cannot move as fully as it once did. Soft tissue around the joint such as muscles and tendons then shorten because they are not used to their full advantage any more. Deformity of the joint often occurs in later stages and can be visible to the naked eye. Have you ever seen someone who is bowlegged? That is one example of a deformity at the knees. Imaging such as x-rays are useful in confirming this diagnosis.

Movement's Impact

Most joints are synovial joints, and this includes joints of the hand, hips, and knees. You may recall we discussed this in Chapter 5. Joints with OA benefit from movement because as the joints move, synovial fluid coats all the bony surfaces. This fluid lubricates the joint and results in less friction, so the ride is smoother if we again use the analogy of a road surface. Synovial fluid provides oxygen and nutrients to the bony surfaces, which helps reduce pain and swelling.

Other purposeful movement including strengthening and stretching can help improve the function of that joint and help normalize the forces within that joint. This allows it to better perform and, therefore, reduces pain and swelling.

There is something to keep in mind here. When you hurt, often the last thing you want to do is move. I get that. But, especially in the early stages of OA, movement is exactly what you need. That's where your physician and movement specialist can help. As I said in Chapter 6, they can assess where you are now and develop a plan to gradually improve your flexibility, strength, and function to reach your goals for the future.

Here's another bonus. Movement can help you lose weight as you begin to burn more calories than you did when you were sitting in pain. Weight loss is a tremendous strategy to help offload those joints where you bear weight like your knees, hips, and even your spine. You will feel better with less down force (or compression) through those joints.

Spinal Stenosis

What Is It?

Certain spine conditions can be considered degenerative, and one of the most common is spinal stenosis. Spinal stenosis is a narrowing of the openings at the side of your spine where the nerves exit from the spinal cord and feed the rest of your body.

Characteristics

Spinal stenosis often occurs at your low back (lumbar spine) and can cause pain down your legs and even numbness and weakness. You can also experience stenosis at the cervical spine (neck). However, this affects your arms and not your legs. The nerves from the spinal cord at the neck feed your arms, and with stenosis, you experience the same symptoms noted above but just at your arms.

Movement's Impact

There is a directional preference for movement with stenosis to help relieve symptoms. It is typically to flex your spine, that is, to bend forward. At your neck, you bring your chin down to your chest. For your low back, just sitting can be enough to relieve your symptoms. Occasionally, you can benefit from sitting at the edge of a chair and bending forward trying to touch your toes. Forward bending enlarges the openings where the nerves go and, therefore, relieves the pressure on those nerves. Standing and arching backward make the openings smaller. This would typically make your symptoms worse.

I cannot stress enough that if you experience these symptoms, please see your physician before trying these maneuvers. They are to be prescribed to you by a trained professional, and you may have certain conditions where bending forward is a risk to you (called a contraindication). Decreased bone density (such as osteopenia and osteoporosis) poses such a risk, for example. Team up with your health professionals to devise a plan that is safe for you. That is why they are there.

Osteoporosis

What Is It?

Osteoporosis is a bone disease that occurs when the body loses too much bone, makes too little bone, or both, according to the National Osteoporosis Foundation (NOF). (NOF, What is Osteoporosis and What Causes It?)

As a result, decreased bone strength and mass significantly increase your risk for fractures. About 54 million Americans have osteoporosis and low bone mass, called osteopenia, and though not as severe as osteoporosis, people with osteopenia are still at increased risk of fracture. A bone density test, called a DEXA scan, can assess bone density at specific body sites and is considered the gold standard for diagnosis. Barring any family history or other comorbidities that may warrant more frequent testing, the NOF recommends women over the age of 65 and men over the age of 70 be tested. Typically, follow-up testing occurs every two to three years and will be determined by your physician.

Characteristics

Unfortunately, osteoporosis is often called a silent disease, because we can't feel our bones weakening. Some are first diagnosed with this disease because of an injury where they sustained a fracture. Others with low bone density often experience pain, especially at the spine, which most write off as occurring due to something else. This is why testing and knowing your numbers are so important.

With advanced stages, a stooped posture is noted and scoliosis can appear as vertebrae compress. Vertebrae and the ends of our long bones such as the femur in the leg and the radius in the arm, are more prone to low bone density because of their composition.

Movement's Impact

Exercise is usually the first line of defense for those with low bone density. Thankfully, you can improve your bone density at any age. The most effective regimen includes weight-bearing exercise such as walking. Impact helps build strong bones, so standing exercises such as marching, can also be beneficial. Core strengthening to protect your spine as well as balance training to reduce risk of falls should also be incorporated into any exercise program. Resistance training also helps, since the bones where muscles and tendons insert get stronger with each lift of a weight.

When you put all of these exercise components together, it becomes a powerful tool to help build strong bones. There are programs designed to do this, but Buff Bones® is one I know very well. I have been a licensed Buff Bones® instructor for almost five years now and have seen the benefits firsthand through my class participants. As a physical therapist, I can get behind the principles of this program, because they are sound and well thought out.

Exercise is often the most desired treatment strategy for bone loss, especially if discovered early. There are medications that can help, but their side effects are not desired by most people. If you have advanced osteoporosis, however, you are likely on some kind of medication dose. Regardless of whether you take medication for this or not, targeted and prescriptive exercise can help.

Diabetes

What Is It?

Diabetes is considered a metabolic disorder that prevents your body from using food properly. Beta cells in the pancreas produce insulin, the hormone that helps blood sugar enter cells to be used as fuel. When you have Type 1 diabetes, beta cells are destroyed by the immune system, so the body doesn't make any insulin. With Type 2 diabetes, beta cells either don't produce enough insulin or the body's cells don't respond to it. Type 2 diabetes most often occurs in adults due to their lifestyle choices.

When blood sugar is unable to penetrate cells to be used for energy, it accumulates in the bloodstream. Over time, the excess blood sugar leads to body-wide damage, including heart and kidney disease, nerve damage, and vision loss. Oral medicines and injectable insulin can help. More importantly, be sure to eat right and move your body.

Characteristics

Diabetes is a very serious condition that you should aggressively manage in partnership with your physician. Examples of damage from this disease include neuropathy (loss of sensation usually to feet and hands), blindness, damage to blood vessels, and amputations. It is critical to control this disease to avoid serious complications, including seizures and even diabetic comas. In the battle against diabetes, a sedentary lifestyle can be your worst enemy. This is why you often see someone with diabetes who is also obese.

Movement's Impact

Prolonged sitting at work, in meetings, or at home watching TV can set back efforts to prevent or manage the disease. The American Diabetes Association (ADA) recommends people with diabetes get up and move for at least three minutes every half hour. According to their evidence-based guidelines, physical movement improves blood sugar management and helps avoid the very high and very low levels of blood sugar. (ADA, Get and Stay Fit)

Exercise helps to lower blood glucose, because it increases insulin sensitivity, your body's ability to use insulin to break down glucose. Insulin sensitivity is heightened during and after physical activity. The more you exercise, the more you help this process.

If you suffer complications from diabetes that make it difficult to exercise, talk to your health provider, such as a physical therapist or physician, about the safest activity for your situation. Keep moving. This is vital for everyone and even more so for those with diabetes.

Two types of physical activity that are most important for managing diabetes are aerobic exercise and strength training, according to the ADA. It adds that if you're not used to being active, you can start with 10 minutes of walking each day and build as your fitness improves.

Dementia

You're probably wondering why I chose to address this one here. If you know me or read my first book, *An Unlikely Gift: Finding Inspiration Caring for My Father with Dementia*, you know that I cared for my dear father for the last 18 years of his life through his battle with dementia. This topic matters to me. What's more, the Centers for Disease Control and Prevention lists Alzheimer's disease (the most common type of dementia) as the sixth leading cause of death in the United States. (CDC, National Center for Health Statistics)

Movement and exercise have an impact on this chronic disease, too.

What Is It?

Dementia is a general term for a decline in mental ability severe enough to interfere with daily life. Memory loss is an example. As noted above, Alzheimer's disease is the most common type of dementia. While the likelihood of having dementia increases with age, it is not a normal part of aging. Light cognitive impairments, such as poorer short-term memory, can happen as a normal part of aging. This is known as age-related cognitive decline rather than dementia, because it does not cause significant problems.

Some risk factors for dementia, such as age and genetics, cannot be changed. But researchers continue to explore the impact of other risk factors on brain health and prevention of dementia. Some of the most active areas of research in risk reduction and prevention include cardiovascular factors, physical fitness, and diet.

Scientists have just recently endorsed three strategies for preventing dementia and cognitive decline associated with normal aging: being physically active, engaging in cognitive training, and controlling high blood pressure.

Characteristics

While symptoms of dementia can vary greatly, at least two of the following core mental functions must be significantly impaired to be considered dementia:

- Memory

- Communication and language

- Ability to focus and pay attention

- Reasoning and judgment

- Visual perception

(Cure Alzheimer's Fund, Dementia)

Movement's Impact

More and more research shows that regular physical exercise may help lower the risk of some types of dementia. It is thought that exercise may directly benefit brain cells by increasing blood and oxygen flow to the brain. Exercise changes the structure and function of the brain as follows:

- Increases brain volume

- Possibly reduces the number and size of age-related holes in the brain's white and gray matter

- Promotes neurogenesis, which is the creation of new brain cells in an already mature brain

Much of the research seems to indicate that aerobic exercise specifically is most effective. Why is this so? According to Gretchen Reynolds of The New York Times, researchers have found that distance running stimulates the release of a particular substance in the brain known as brain-derived neurotrophic factor (BDNF) that is known to regulate neurogenesis. The more miles an animal runs, the more BDNF it produces. (Reynolds, Gretchen, Exercise Best for the Brain)

Some evidence suggests it's never too late to start exercising for brain health. According to Alzheimer's & Dementia, a study at the University of Eastern Finland found that physical activities in midlife seem to protect from dementia in old age. Researchers found that participants who engaged in physical activities at least two times per week had a lower risk of dementia than those who were less active. (Alzheimer's & Dementia, Physical Activity)

More research is under way, but based on what we know so far, we can surmise that what is good for the heart (aerobic exercise) is also good for the brain. Start early. Start now.

To summarize, movement is medicine, and it couldn't be more true for those with chronic conditions that occur as we age. Movement can help them all. For even more good news, you don't need to walk this road alone. In fact, always consult with your physician about your condition and when starting any new exercise program. Request a referral to a physical or occupational therapist to help gently and safely guide you to a more active lifestyle. These are lifestyle choices and your choices now will define your future.

Here's another key to all this movement talk. Many of my patients do not like taking prescription medications. They don't want to rely on them or worse get addicted to them. They don't like the side effects, especially constipation, which is not only painful but dangerous. Movement and prescriptive exercise that you get from a therapist can effectively reduce the medications you take. Keep moving and you may not need that pill you take.

This is powerful, my friends, and you have the ability–yes, you, and only you–to make this happen. Now that should get your attention. Health is wealth. Are you ready to get rich?

Chapter 8 Invest in Yourself

If you're reading this book, chances are you are in your midlife, say somewhere between age 40 to 60 (or beyond). Hopefully, you have some money saved up for your next phase of life or retirement. Call it what you will. Personally, I like to call it my next phase. The word retirement to me is kicking back, putting my feet up, and relaxing. Sure, I may want to do that from time to time, but I want my next phase to be active, and I want to be with active people as much as possible. I want to travel and visit family and friends in faraway places. I want to golf. I want to get better at playing pickleball and maybe learn another sport I haven't considered yet. I want to do something.

How did you go about saving for your next phase? Do you have a pension? Do you have a retirement account? What other ways did you invest and save your money? Why did you do that? Why did you forego spending the money you were earning at the time? Why did you tell your employer to take a percentage of your earnings out of your paycheck and put it into your 401(k)? Why? I suspect you did it to invest in your future. You did it to help make your future years on Earth enjoyable and fulfilling, right? You did it so you could perhaps travel and spend time with loved ones. You did it to celebrate this part of your life. Did you use that same discipline and effort to invest in your health so you could have the physical capacity to do these things?

Think of movement as investing in your future. Every time you move, every time you exercise, you are putting money in your body bank. You are building up your savings to do the things you want to do. You are investing in your body to make your next years your best years. Your physical health is like money in the bank. It enables you to do the things you want to do with your life.

Movement is functional. Movement is life. Move, and remember the returns will make you rich. Rich in terms of filling each day with activities you enjoy and being with people who mean the world to you. Rich in terms of living freely and independently. Wealth is freedom to do what you want. You benefit twice. You reap rewards of the activity itself, and you benefit later from having a strong and fit body.

There is more good news. You can start any time. It doesn't matter where you're at right now. We each have our own starting point. Respect it and move on. Make a plan. Did you make a financial plan for your life? I bet most of you did. Why not make a plan and maybe even consult with a specialist to help steer you in the proper direction? Your future is worth it, right?

Well, the same applies to your physical health. Are you collaborating with your physician to improve your health? Often, we are so reactive. We only consult our physician when something goes wrong. How about working with your physician and other healthcare providers to build a plan to make things right? How about creating a plan to make your body as strong as possible for your future dreams? This makes sense, doesn't it? Why not schedule this type of visit with your physician or movement specialist right now?

Do you have a cash reserve fund? In other words, do you have an emergency fund in case something happens and you need cash now? Maybe there was a bad storm and damage to your home requires immediate attention. Worse yet, maybe there were layoffs where you work and you lose your job. Maybe a pandemic sweeps the country and you are furloughed for months or more. (I know. Crazy, right?) You can't possibly know everything that's coming your way. You want to be prepared so you can help protect you and your family. A cash reserve helps build up your resources so you can better manage the hard times and recover more quickly and easily.

The same applies to your reserves of physical health. We learned earlier that our bodies change as we age. Our environment and even our genes may not be kind to us. Accidents happen, too, don't they? We can get injured by unexpected falls or car accidents and in other ways. One diagnosis can put you into a tailspin. Perhaps you might even need surgery to correct an ailment. Things happen. Life happens.

By moving and exercising, you are building your health reserves. A more fit person will recover faster and more fully than an unhealthy one. I have seen it over and over again. And this is regardless of age. The stronger you are going into an injury or sickness, the better you will be coming out of it. The same applies for surgery. That is why many facilities offer what some call *prehab* before a planned surgery. This is very common for those with a scheduled hip or knee replacement. By improving range of motion and strength before surgery (hence the term prehab), you greatly increase your chance of a better outcome after surgery. Build your reserves now for your body bank.

Here is another example of why I ask you to start moving now. I mentioned before that as I write this, we are in the midst of the most serious pandemic of our lives. Lives are lost on a daily basis due to this disease. Let our times teach you. Are you one pandemic away from an early death? Are you one fall or injury away from not returning to the home you love? Are you one surgery away from living in a facility the rest of your life?

Sorry to be blunt. This is tough. But how close are you? Do you live alone in a multistory home? If so, have you been up to the second floor in the past year? It was not unusual for me to have patients who have not been upstairs in their own home in years. They don't even remember what is up there. Have you fallen recently? Are you avoiding going out shopping due to fear? Are family members or paid help getting your groceries and your medicine? Do you have prepared meals delivered? Please know I am not judging you here. These are the very things that are available so you can remain in your home. I get it. Just know that if it gets to this point, you're getting closer.

Realize, too, that if something were to happen and you are admitted to the hospital, you will need to meet the hospital's standards of safety in order to return home. If you don't, they may suggest you continue your recovery at a skilled nursing facility where you will participate in physical, occupational, and even speech therapy. Here you can continue to improve your strength, mobility, and balance so you can ultimately return home safely. Hopefully, you are able to return home, but know that some people don't. This can be a very difficult time.

Are you willing to let others make choices about where you should live because you were only one step away? If you're like me and many others, the polite answer is no, you don't want to live that close. Here's my real response to that question–hell no.

My recommendation is to make choices now that serve you. Be intentional with your life. Get in that driver's seat. Drive the bus that is your life. Honk your horn every chance you get. Invest in yourself, and do it now. The more we invest in ourselves over time, the richer our lives will be. Move like your life depends on it, because it does.

Your time is precious. Be good to yourself. Every time I work out, I consider it my time. Life is busy. I get it. But how cool is this? By dedicating one hour of your time per day, three times per week (or whatever you choose it to be), you are honoring yourself. Nobody else. You have decided to dedicate that time to something precious—you. Sometimes I don't feel like exercising. There, I said it. It's true. But I do it. And oftentimes, I do it for me, to be with just me. This is my hour—no one else's. It's good for the soul folks. If you're like me, you can use this time to recharge you, calm you, center you, ground you. Let it be whatever you need at the moment. You do so many things for other people, and you likely do this every day. Take just a fraction of that time for you. It's not selfish. It's necessary. This is truly one of the best ways to invest in yourself.

Your body is precious. Treat it as such. I learned the following concept when I became a physical therapist. We spent years in school to learn about certain conditions, diseases, and injuries and then to develop a plan to help you recover and, hopefully, resume your normal life. I learned what exercises were best for someone with a knee replacement, a rotator cuff tear, and many things in between. I know how many repetitions you should do and how often you should perform them. I know signs and symptoms to look out for when things don't go right and can guide you through these things. Giving someone an exercise to do is easy.

But I quickly learned what was more important. I am here to give you the tools to get your life back. I am here to help rid you of the pain you've had for much too long. I am here to help you return to work. I am here to help you play with your grandchildren. I am here to help you walk down the aisle at your daughter's wedding (true more than once). I am here to help you go on and enjoy your dream vacation. Feel free to fill in the blank here. There are so many more very good reasons to move. Movement is more than just an activity or exercise. Movement is the means for your dreams.

I often never know the final outcome for someone I treated as a therapist or fitness professional. But sometimes, I do.

> "Personally, I have to say that meeting you changed my life. I came to you with one problem that developed over a few months after my heel spur surgery. Only a few sessions into therapy and I fractured vertebrae falling through a stairway. Resuming PT, you worked with me on both problems and more. Well prior to the heel and back, I had been suffering from varying degrees of sciatica for about 5 years. Chiropractic sessions and my inversion table helped me manage it but it never went away. Since we parted in early May, 2019, I have not experienced ANY sciatic bouts. Last September I was doing some sidewalk repair and that included many trips to the hardware store for numerous (about 20) 80-pound bags of concrete mix which I carried on my shoulder. I was indeed tired at the end of each day, but absolutely NO leg/back pain.
>
> Honestly, a year ago, I had nearly accepted the thought that I would be living with pain for the rest of my years. I don't mean to sound dramatic, but all the above is true. THANK YOU again." Brian R.

This gentleman had pain for years and thought he always would. He made the investment and it paid off. I'm giving you more than just an exercise. I'm trying to give you your life back. Movement can bring you your life back. Movement can take away your pain. It did for Brian, and it did for me when I hurt my back in college. Movement and exercise are so much more than meets the eye. This is your body we're talking about. This is your investment.

Activity #3

Time to take this into your own hands. Please revisit your journal and get ready to add the next section to your action plan. Title this one *Assessment and Goals*.

Reflect on what you have written so far. What have you learned? Has one thing stood out that is really burning inside you? What is your repeated self-talk? When you look at your strengths, what tools do you have to take your life forward? What do you want?

I want you now to reflect on your activity level of late. Are you more active or less active? If you're less active, what activities have been dropped from your life? Why? Do you want to resume them again? Is there a new activity or sport that interests you? Would this new activity help you get out of the house and meet new people if that is your desire?

You may have this in place now due to your journaling above, but I want you to identify 10 things you want to do, be or have. These should be achievable and meaningful to you. Write down whatever comes to mind. Just let it flow. We'll discuss these again soon. Ten things–go.

Chapter 9 You Can Live Well

"I just wanted you to know that my back is better than it has been in years. I faithfully do my PT routine you constructed for me at least every other day gradually increasing the reps and have stuck to that since our last appointment, a year ago in March 2019. You have helped me do what several other doctors and specialists have failed to do and I am forever grateful." Scott K.

Never, ever give up. Never.

You can live well. Please rethink your expectations. Please consider there might be another way. Please just try.

One of the biggest questions I get from my patients and clients is, "Where do I start? What should I do?" These are very valid questions and the unknown can seem like a barrier. Some of you are hurting, haven't moved in a very long time (in some cases years), or have very limited tolerance to movement as a result of your health. Often, you have all of these (and more) to contend with and overcome. You're scared. You want to move, but you don't want to feel worse. I get it. We'll start at the beginning.

My goal for this chapter is to give you some ideas about where to start. First, however, I must say that you should always consult with your physician before you start any new exercise program. Second, consult with movement professionals such as physical therapists and occupational therapists who can skillfully evaluate you and then suggest appropriate exercises for you to do based on your goals. Go to other trusted professionals who know you and your body and who can advise you as to how to start.

The key is to just start. Make the call. A gentleman in one of my specialized fitness classes posed this question to me once and it instantly made me appreciate the challenges some people have. He asked what his wife should do to start moving. "Tell me more about her health and activity level," I asked. He responded, "She sits in a chair all day long. The only time she gets up is to use the bathroom and get something to eat. That's it. Day after day." Once he shared this, I asked when she saw her physician last. He said he wasn't sure but guessed about six months ago. I quickly remarked that before she starts anything, she should get clearance from her physician to start. "Would it be appropriate for her to join me in this class?" he asked. "No," I said. Given her history of a sedentary lifestyle, I knew that this class would be too strenuous for her. This class included a full hour of exercise with position changes and resistance training with weights. It required keeping a certain pace along with the rest of the class. It was just too much to ask of her. A more appropriate start would be for her to consult with her physician and request a referral to physical therapy.

I have treated many patients just like his wife. As long as she was medically stable and her physical exam revealed a potential to benefit from therapy, a simple progression from seated to standing exercises might be appropriate. She could start with simple exercises to move her arms and legs with some repetition involved. Some of my patients can start with performing five repetitions, and some are able to perform 20 reps. Both are just fine. Respect the starting point, right? Lifting a body part up toward the ceiling can be enough work for someone. Using gravity as resistance can be very effective.

Alternatively, I have seen the above program be too much for some people. It either exhausts them, or they cannot perform it safely. If that is the case, another option is to just walk. For the gentleman's wife above, this is an activity that we know she can do. She already does it. She could start by just doing it more frequently during the day. Then she could progress to walking longer each time. This is functional movement at its purest form. I know it's not glamorous, but it is so important. Walking longer and more frequently will help you tolerate appointments and events out of the home better and maybe you could stop at the store on your way home to pick up a few things. That's huge for some folks.

I have given the recommendation to walk more to many homecare patients at my very first visit with them. No exercises are given yet. I just ask them to walk more in their home—how far and how often depend on their current status. That is their homework and their only homework until I see them again. Walking is a fabulous exercise. Walking works on flexibility, strength, endurance, and balance training all at once. It works on multiple systems in the body including the musculoskeletal system, the cardiovascular system, respiratory system, and even our immune system. Talk about getting your bang for your buck. Now that's a smart investment.

Walking is just one example of an effective way to get started. There are more examples that I want to share with you to help you move. As a physical therapist treating thousands of patients over the years, I have learned what movements work well for those with certain conditions. Be sure, not everyone is the same and not everyone responds the same way to certain exercises. but what I have learned is that there are trends of success for those with certain diagnoses. Soon, I will reveal some very basic exercises that have worked for a large majority of my patients. But first, I want to help you understand your starting point.

My goal here is to get and keep you moving safely. To that end, you have things to consider:

- How active are you now?

- What hurts? Can you embrace the notion that movement can help you feel better?

- How is your overall health? What conditions do you manage and how will exercise impact them?

- What is important to you? What kind of lifestyle do you want? What do you want to be able to do that you currently can't do—or can't do well?

- What health conditions do you want to avoid? Maybe a family member has experienced something that you don't want. Can exercise help that?

- How can you live well, feel good, and have the energy you want to do the things you enjoy?

The answers to these questions can really tap into your motivation and deep desires. Don't just breeze over them. Take some time and live with them for a while. Add these answers to what you already have in your journal from your last activity in Chapter 8, Assessment and Goals. I told you we'd get to them soon. What gets your attention. What do you keep going back to? That desire can lead to the level of intent you need to make a change in your life. Write about it. Live it for a while. Imagine every last detail of your ideal life. Think of it this way: Don't ask if you are worthy of your goal or goals. Ask if your goals are worthy of you. They must serve you. If they don't, move on to those that do. At this time, please identify the top three things you want to do, be, or have. We'll revisit them a little later.

I've spent a lot of time thinking about how to organize my movement and exercise recommendations so that they mean something to you. I call on my years of experience as a physical therapist to help me here. I think of my patients and what has motivated so many of them. What worked for them? What are the things they continued to work on years after we worked together? I've had the privilege to see some of my patients I've worked with before, and I smile when I see they have the same paper of exercises I gave them way back then. The pages are often pretty beat up, but they have them and use them still. Remember Scott K? He still has his. We do what works.

Without meeting each and every one of you who are reading this book, I want to do my best to give you what works and to help you be successful. There are some common traits to start this process, and they have to do with identifying what your activity level is now. I use three classifications for this. See which one best describes you.

Sedentary

- You sit at least 75 percent of the day. This may even be in only one or two chairs in your home.

- You don't leave your home except for appointments or to shop with family or friends.

- You may only get out of your chair to make a meal and/or use the bathroom. If your bedroom is on another floor, you don't go back there until it's time for bed, or you may decide to stay where you are (in your chair or recliner) and sleep there.

- You have everything you need all around you at one main chair. One table has the phone, remote for the TV, pen and paper, and maybe a tablet or iPad. The other table has today's newspaper, magazines, mail that needs your attention, and perhaps a pill organizer box labeled with days of the week.

- Typically, you have pain and stiffness, so you do not want to move any more than necessary.

Active

- You sit between 40 to 60 percent of the day.

- You might be retired or work at a desk much of the day. Maybe you volunteer. You might leave your home two to four days each week and regularly meet friends, go out to eat, or attend a social function.

- Sometimes when you sit, you sit for a long time. Activity comes in bunches.

- Energy level is not what it used to be. Once you're moving, you feel grateful you did it, but getting to that point can be difficult.

Very Active

- You sit less than 30 percent of the day.

- You are out of the home most days of the week. Perhaps you work or volunteer regularly.

- Maybe you participate in athletic pursuits on a consistent basis such as golf, hiking, biking, tennis, or pickleball.

- You are social and enjoy being with others.

As you can see, there are some gray areas between these segments, but they are three distinct lifestyles. Perhaps you drift from one to another over the course of time. I suggest making your starting point by picking a segment where you spend most of your time, say in the last six to nine months.

Here's what isn't gray. Did you notice my first criteria for each segment was how often you sit? Nothing about sitting still in a chair is active. I know this seems pretty obvious, but it's worth discussing. Sitting is static and not favorable for good health. Sure, we can't stand and walk all day long. There needs to be a balance and the balance for most healthy individuals should be that they sit less. Maybe you've heard the saying, "Sitting is the new smoking." I don't know who first said it, but I believe it completely and I believe it is a barometer for your health.

I also want to point something else out here. This is a no judgment zone. By that I mean I realize there are other factors that can lead you down a path to less activity and, quite frankly, less motivation. Do you work? If so, do you primarily sit all day? If you do, do you find a way to move when you're not working? Do you exercise early in the day before you go to work? Can you take a walk either inside your building or outside of it during your lunch break? If you're not an early bird, are you active after work by exercising or taking a walk? You must make time to move to counterbalance all that sitting time.

Another effective strategy to decrease pain and stiffness when sitting during the day is to take what I call microbreaks. If possible, time it. Say, every half hour, stand up and do a lap around your home or office. Maybe walk to the restroom (even if you don't have to go). Visit a colleague elsewhere in the office. Do something to get out of that seated position. This can also be a great strategy to help improve your posture when seated. This is addressed in detail in Chapter 10.

Now, guess what, it's time for you to take a microbreak. Do you know how long you've been seated reading this book? Go ahead, get up and take a walk around your home or even outside. It's time. We'll see you on the other side.

———

Now don't you feel better? More aware and more alert. Keep up the great work. I actually have a fitness watch that tells me to get up if I'm sitting too long. If I can't stand, it even gives me seated activities to do in place of it. This might occur during a long car ride, for example. I listen to it and follow it every time. It matters. I offer it as an idea for you to consider.

Work and life events aside, our environment also plays a huge role in our activity level. What is your home like? Is it big or is it small? How many rooms do you have? Do you have stairs inside? If so, how many flights? Do you have steps outside to negotiate before you even get to the door? Is there a handrail at any of them? Do you have a sidewalk outside your home or is it an uneven grass or gravel surface? Does it slope down, up, or sideways? Could you go outside regularly and take a walk? Could you do it safely?

Where do you live? Is it winter outside six months of the year? Do you get a lot of snow and ice? Are you high on a hill where the wind can really howl and maybe even knock you over? Don't laugh. I visited a patient's home in the Finger Lakes once that was on top of Italy Hill. Have you heard of that? It has one of the highest elevations in the area at just over 1600 feet. It is open farm land primarily, and oh how that wind can blow up there. Combine that with snow at that elevation and it is downright nasty. I once treated a woman who lived on this hill–in the middle of winter. She was in her late 60s, lived alone, and was recovering from a total knee replacement. I think you need to be tough to live in that kind of environment, and she was, and she had a lot of friends. One neighbor made sure her driveway was plowed for the likes of me, other healthcare professionals, and friends who visited her. Another friend made meals and brought them over to her every so often. Neighbors got together and hand delivered her mail to her so she didn't have to walk down her long driveway to get it. Using a walker, with a limp, in conditions as described above, is just not safe.

She recovered well, but I hope you get the picture. Environment can work for or against you and can make a big difference in how active you are. It can also make a big difference in your ability to exercise. I once worked with a man in his second-floor apartment that was one of the smallest I had ever seen, and it was also extremely cluttered. To be clear, he didn't have a lot of extra furniture and objects that were extraneous. He lived modestly and had a sectional couch and dining room table in one room. He had a bed and dresser in another room, and he had a small kitchen that you could walk into and then quickly out of with three large steps. There were no straight paths in the room where the couch and dining room table were located. He and I had to side step to move about in there. There was not enough room for him to use his walker that he needed when he first got home after surgery. There was no place to exercise effectively. Did I mention he had to climb 19 steps outside of the home to get to his apartment? I saw him because he had just had a knee replacement. He did the best he could despite his surroundings.

Think about your environment, and identify the pros and cons to movement there. How can you keep moving with what you have? Some people actually move to improve their accessibility and their safety. You've heard of downsizing, right? Many older adults move to a home where everything is on one floor. Doorways are wide enough to accommodate someone in a wheelchair if necessary. Cabinets are at a lower height for easy reach. Many folks become snowbirds or downright move from northern to southern climates, so they can be more active and outside throughout the year. (I wonder who that could be.)

Think about where you are and how you want your life to be in 5 to 10 years. What does it look like? Where is it? How does it make you feel? Come up with some options that appeal to you and your family. There are always options. Jot these down in your journal.

Regardless of where you are, do what you can to be active now. It may mean marching in place in the living room or kitchen if space is limited. You can always do something. My gentleman patient in the small apartment could repeatedly sit in his dining room chair and then stand as one of his exercises to work on his strength, range of motion, and balance. Not to mention he was getting very good at something he does in real life every day. Don't say, "I can't because." Say instead, "How can I? How can I move more with what I have?"

How can you? I am going to show you how. I asked you earlier to define your activity level. That, for the sake of this discussion, is your starting point. Remember, be true to where you are. Own it. Next, I will use two parameters to define your destination. I choose these as I have found them to repeatedly mean the most to the thousands of patients I have treated over the years.

Please take a look now at the goals you wrote at the end of Chapter 8 and then later defined earlier in this chapter. Keep them in your sights as you continue reading here. Your goals are personal to you, and I want you to hold on to them. Do they have anything in common with what I'm about to share? The two parameters or most overarching themes I hear are:

"I want to improve my mobility and my balance."

"I want to decrease my pain and stiffness (from arthritis)."

Do any of your goals reflect something similar? They might be worded differently. Here are some of the responses I hear almost every day:

"I want my independence."

"I want to enjoy activities again with increased strength and energy."

"I want less pain."

"I want to feel good again."

Please look at your goals and find some common ground. Chance are good you already know what that is. What is your why? Do you want to keep up with your spouse? Do you want to be able to play with your grandkids? Do you want to go on that fabulous vacation to Europe? Do you want to keep playing sports?

What Is Your Why?

There are so many different ways people want to spend their second half of life. What do you all have in common? You need to move and be mobile enough to achieve what you want. You need to get up. There is no magic wand, and there is no magic pill to make the gains you want. I once did a search online on how to treat arthritis. The first results were pills that can cure you of arthritis. Be pain free in five days was just one of the claims. No, no, no. There is no cure for arthritis. There are no magic cures for the chronic conditions that ail you unless you consider movement as magic. Now, you're onto something.

The following chart summarizes what we've discussed so far from where you are now down to where you want to be.

Goals		
Activity Level	**Walk More with Better Balance**	**Decrease Pain and Stiffness**
Sedentary	How can I?	How can I?
Active	How can I?	How can I?
Very active	How can I?	How can I?

The question becomes, "How can I walk more and have better balance?" The answers (or the how) will be different for those of you who are sedentary than they would be if you were active or very active. The answers would also be different for each activity level when we ask the question, "How can I decrease my pain and stiffness?"

What is interesting here is that once you start to move more, you move down to the next activity level. There, you meet up with different exercises and movements to better match your new health status at the time. So, those of you who were once sedentary now become active. If you keep moving and get stronger and more mobile, you can ultimately progress to being very active. Your needs and likely your interests will change over time. As a physical therapist, this is a beautiful thing to watch. But it's an even greater thing for you to experience.

Everyone has a starting place. You already defined that. Now, I want you to pick one of the goals above that is most closely aligned with your top three goals. Which one matters the most to you right now? You may want to consider which one is most doable for you right now. That is, you may want to decrease your pain and stiffness first to allow you to walk more and do it more comfortably. In this case, achieving the first goal sets you up for success for the second goal.

By picking one of the goals above now, you will be able to clearly see what should happen next. As you continue to read this book, the goal you just picked will guide you down a specific path. I will lay out for you in the next chapter action items to help you achieve your goal based on your activity level.

So, right now, identify your activity level (your starting point) as sedentary, active, or very active.

Then, choose one of the goals below (your destination) that matters most to you right now:

"I want to improve my mobility and my balance."

"I want to decrease my pain and stiffness."

Perfect. Your navigator is set. You have mapped out your route. Trips can be so much fun. Time to go. Let's do this.

Chapter 10 Go Time

So here we go. It's time to take action. This chapter is structured to help you first see the bigger picture of your new life and then funnel it down from there. Later, we will drill down to specific activities and exercises you should do to help you reach your goal. The following recommendations are organized by your current fitness level, and each section describes your activities for one week. Please review this now by referencing your current fitness level.

Sedentary		
Day	**Activities**	**Duration**
Monday	Aerobic training	5-10 minutes
	Exercise	15-20 minutes
Wednesday	Movement (your choice)	15-30 minutes
Friday	Aerobic training	5-10 minutes
	Exercise	15-20 minutes
Saturday	Movement (your choice)	15-30 minutes
Active		
Day	**Activities**	**Duration**
Monday	Aerobic training	15-30 minutes
	Exercise	15-30 minutes
Wednesday	Movement (your choice)	30-60 minutes
Friday	Aerobic training	15-30 minutes
	Exercise	15-30 minutes
Saturday	Movement (your choice)	30-60 minutes

Very Active		
Day	**Activities**	**Duration**
Monday	Aerobic training	35-45 minutes
	Exercise	15-30 minutes
Wednesday	Movement (your choice)	60+ minutes
Friday	Aerobic training	35-45 minutes
	Exercise	15-30 minutes
Saturday	Movement (your choice)	60+ minutes

I designed these recommendations for you with the following in mind:

- The time devoted to any activity increases with your fitness level.

- Sessions are structured to not exceed one hour as research shows anything more than this is less likely to be continued over time.

- Activities occur four days a week, so you are active for the majority of the week.

- Monday, Wednesday, Friday, and Saturday are arbitrary. Feel free to pick your own days of the week to fit your needs and lifestyle. Try not to schedule these activities on consecutive days if you are just starting out or if you have been aggressive in your movement.

- Duration ranges of time are provided to allow for your own fitness level and desires.

As you can see, activities are separated into categories including aerobic training, movement, and exercise. The following describes these in more detail to help you identify what is appropriate for you to do for each.

Aerobic Training

This includes any activity sustained over time that will raise your heart rate for cardiovascular training. The term *aerobic* means you use oxygen continuously. This is also called *cardio* exercise and may include:

- Walking (on pavement or treadmill)

- Bicycling (over the road or stationary)

- Using equipment in a fitness center such as an elliptical or a rowing machine

- Any program designed for cardiovascular exercise (class or video)

Keep In Mind

Start slow and build up your exertion level over time, especially if you are sedentary.

Continue reading this chapter and see Appendix B for specific guidelines for proper exercise intensity.

Use the talk test. You should be able to talk and complete at least one full sentence without shortness of breath during this activity.

Movement

Movement can include household activities such as cleaning, meal prep and cooking, gardening, lawn care, and walking the dog. Movement can include recreational activities like hiking, biking, etc. Quite honestly, the options here are endless. You can even do varied activities and add the time up to equal your total time for movement in a day.

Keep in Mind

- Is it doable? Do you have the environment to do it safely?

- Is it meaningful for you?

- Can your family participate with you? Or do you want to be by yourself?

- Is it fun? Is it something that helps you feel satisfied and fulfilled?

- Does it make you smile? Does it make you laugh?

- Can you easily repeat it on a regular basis? For example, is it a recreational activity such as golf or pickleball that you can participate on a daily or weekly basis?

Movement can take so many forms. Maybe you have a home project you want to start. Perfect. That counts. Maybe you really need to get out there and tend to your garden. Yes, that counts, too. What ideas do you have to help you move today?

Exercise

Remember that exercise is a form of movement. And exercise that has meaning and is relevant to your goals is called prescriptive exercise. Many of you may be willing to try some structured and meaningful exercise to reach your goals. What follows will provide ways to effectively do that.

The following table expands on what we started in the previous chapter. It identifies movement and exercises to do for each fitness level and goal. Some are self-explanatory. Many are more fully described in Appendix A. Please review this Appendix in detail.

As stated earlier, always consult with your physician before starting any new exercise program. Take this book to help you share your ideas and goals. Consider a referral to a physical therapist for a more customized program to meet your needs in a safe manner. (Please refer to the Limit of Liability/Disclaimer of Warranty in the front of this book for additional information.)

Below are activities that respect your starting point and can help you achieve your goal. These meet your needs for flexibility, strengthening, and endurance as well as gait and balance training. These are just a sample of the type of movements appropriate for any given level. This is not an exhaustive list by any *stretch* (pun intended). Consider this a starting point. Some exercises appear for both goals. This is not a mistake. They can help achieve either goal. This shows how one exercise can be beneficial to you in multiple ways. Movement is a miracle.

So, let's drill down into each category based on your activity level and goal.

Activity Level	Walk More with Better Balance	Decrease Pain and Stiffness
Sedentary	Walk more frequently	Walk more frequently
	Walk longer	Walk longer
	Seated exercises Legs • Heel raises • Marches • Kickouts Arms • Rows • Bicep curls • Punches	Seated exercises Legs • Heel raises • Marches • Kickouts Arms • Rows • Bicep curls • Punches
	Standing exercises • Heel/toe raises • Marches • Hip abduction • Hip abduction	Supine (lying) • Heel slides • Quad sets • Glut sets • Ankle pumps
Active	Walk longer outside or gym	Walk longer outside or gym
	Seated/standing exercises with weights	Add stretching • Calf • Hamstring • Knee to chest
	Add seated clam with band	

Activity Level	Walk More with Better Balance	Decrease Pain and Stiffness
	Squats Static balance training • Wide to narrow BOS • Eyes open to eyes closed • Single leg stance	Continue supine exercises • Add straight leg raise • Add pelvic tilts • Add tabletop foot taps • Add clam with band
Very active	Walk longer regularly	Walk longer regularly
	Core strengthening	Core strengthening .
	Planks	Planks
	Dynamic balance training • Side stepping • Walking forward and back • Sit to stand to sit	Continue stretching
	Sporting activity	Sporting activity

Please visit Appendix A now to learn more about each prescriptive exercise listed above. Here you will see each exercise listed alphabetically with a written description as to how to perform each one and organized by strengthening exercises, stretching exercises, and balance training. You will learn more about balance training in the next chapter, so stay tuned for that.

Keep in mind that once you start to move more and increase your activity level, you will be asked to perform different exercises and movements that match your new health status at the time. This is fluid and dynamic in nature. Your fitness level, activities, and likely your interests will change over time. For that reason alone, please hold onto this book, because life will change and likely your goals will change, too. Pick up this book anytime and follow it along the path to action and reward, regardless of your starting point.

Frequency, Duration, and Intensity

Now that we have all this content, let's talk about how to structure your activities. One of the most commons questions I hear is, "How many do I do, and how often should I do them?" Great question.

When I'm working with someone in the rehab setting who may have just had surgery, I might start with 10 reps of a certain movement and ask my patient to perform them twice per day except for therapy days. Eventually, once discharged from therapy, I ask my patients to perform certain movements three to four times per week to maintain what they have. This is consistent with the weekly schedule I proposed earlier in this chapter.

The number of repetitions you do depends on your activity level. For someone sedentary, you may start with 5 to 10 reps and work up from there. Someone who is active may be able to perform 10 to 20 reps at a time safely. Always know that repetitions and resistance are closely related. To get stronger, you must increase your resistance over time. This is discussed in more detail in Chapter 12. Your resistance is how much weight you are moving, which is proportional to the force you need to provide. The following table shows a reasonable start to your program.

Activity Level	Starting Repetitions	Starting Resistance
Sedentary	5-10	Gravity only with no added resistance
Active	10-20	Gravity to light resistance
Very active	20-30	Light to moderate resistance

For strengthening exercises, I use a rule of 30 to define the right progression. If you can perform 30 reps without fatigue with good form while using a certain weight, then add a pound or two of weight. You may not be able to perform 30 repetitions with the added resistance, but do what you can safely and work up to 30 over time. Don't be fooled by the impact gravity can have on your activity or exercise. Gravity acts as a downward force when lifting any part of your body up and can be challenging for any of you. Respect it. Start light and work on learning the desired movement. Then you can add more resistance based on the guidelines provided here.

For the record, I don't increase stretching repetitions or holds over time. These will remain the same, though if you wanted to do a certain stretch more than the recommendation, that is an option for you.

Our government defines global standards for exercise and I include them here for your reference. The U.S. Department of Health and Human Services recommends the following exercise guidelines for healthy adults to follow as it relates to frequency, duration, and intensity. (U.S. Department of Health and Human Services, Physical Activity Guidelines for Americans)

- Aerobic activity: Get at least 150 minutes of moderate activity or 75 minutes of vigorous activity per week. You can also perform an equivalent combination of moderate- and vigorous-intensity aerobic activity. It's also okay to break things up. For example, you'll get there by exercising for 30 minutes, 5 times a week.

- Additional health benefits are gained by engaging in physical activity beyond the equivalent of 300 minutes of moderate-intensity physical activity a week.

- Adults should also do muscle-strengthening activities of moderate or greater intensity and that involve all major muscle groups two or more days a week, as these activities provide additional health benefits.

The key guidelines for adults also apply to older adults. In addition, the following key guidelines are for older adults:

- As part of their weekly physical activity, older adults should do multicomponent physical activity that includes balance training as well as aerobic and muscle-strengthening activities.

- Older adults should determine their level of effort for physical activity relative to their level of fitness.

- Older adults with chronic conditions should understand whether and how their conditions affect their ability to do regular physical activity safely.

- When older adults cannot do 150 minutes of moderate-intensity aerobic activity a week because of chronic conditions, they should be as physically active as their abilities and conditions allow.

For those adults with chronic conditions who cannot meet the above guidelines, consider these recommendations:

- Engage in regular physical activity according to your abilities. Avoid inactivity.

- If you have one or more chronic conditions, please consult with a healthcare professional or physical activity specialist about the types and amounts of activity appropriate for your abilities and chronic conditions.

Intensity is another factor to consider when you exercise. There are general guidelines to follow and I've outlined the most common in Appendix B. Again, if you have one or more chronic condition, please consult with your healthcare provider for guidelines you should follow based on your specific health history.

As you start to move more and become more active, please keep the following in mind.

Drink Plenty of Water

Your body performs best when it's properly hydrated. Failing to drink enough water when you are exerting yourself over a prolonged period of time, especially in hot conditions, can be dangerous. Many organizations recommend drinking 64 fluid ounces of water a day. I recommend you take that further and add to that amount replacement fluids for coffee, tea, or alcohol you consume that day. These drinks are considered to be diuretic in nature as they increase the amount of water removed from the body in the form of urine. To be sure you're hydrated properly, consider also adding more water for every hour of exercise. This could amount to an extra 16 to 24 ounces of water per day depending on how much you perspire.

I bet it sounds like a lot to you. It did to me at first, too. But it helps tremendously. I drink at least 80 oz. of water per day. My body now depends on it. On active days, I consumer over 100 oz. Why? Because I feel better. My energy is higher. I am more fit and I can more easily control my weight. I could write a whole chapter about water and its health benefits. It is important to note that most people, especially adults over 65, spend much of their time dehydrated. It is one of the most common reasons for hospitalization for older adults. It can also be deadly. And it can so easily be prevented. Drink more water.

Please note certain medical conditions may require you to limit your fluid intake, including, among other diagnoses, congestive heart failure. Please consult with your physician to know your specific guidelines to follow.

Listen to Your Body

If you feel pain or discomfort while working out, stop. If you feel better after a brief rest, you can slowly and gently resume your workout, but don't try to power through pain. That's a recipe for injury.

There is good pain and there is bad pain. I'll start with the bad pain. This is what to avoid. This is pain produced at a joint that is not easily relieved. This is the pain you want to get rid of and may be why you're exercising in the first place. Good pain is muscle soreness (not at a joint) that is produced typically a day after a new exercise or activity is introduced. It typically lasts 24 to 48 hours and then slowly dissipates. This is called delayed onset muscle soreness and is a sign you are getting stronger. Good pain should be monitored, but is not a reason to stop the activity. Bad pain is reason to stop the activity. If that should occur, please consult with your physician to help diagnose the issue and come up with a solution.

Reminder: Please consult with your physician before starting any new exercise program. Your physician knows the details of your past medical history and current status to advise you properly. Perhaps take this book with you to your visit and show your physician what you are considering. That will greatly help him or her work with you to help define your starting point. This should be a team effort.

Form Matters

Physical therapy training and experience have taught me that form is very important. I define form as the position your body is in while performing an activity such as the exercises noted in this book. It is about joint angles and the length/tension relationships of soft tissue in the body.

Alternatively, you have likely heard of the term, posture, such as in the sentence, "Sit up tall, you're slouching." Form is similar to posture. I will use the term, form, to describe proper positioning during exercise. However, please take the time to review Appendix C that discusses posture in more detail and further identifies what proper posture is in our everyday life.

I wish I could see you move, but I can't. I can't cue you to keep your knees behind your toes, for example. I can't cue you to narrow your stance if needed for a balance challenge. Good form addresses your needs. It decreases your pain. Wrong form can cause your pain to continue or even worsen. At the very least, poor form means that you are not doing what is intended with the activity. It may not hurt you, but it's just not doing what we mean it to do. That's when a movement professional can help you. We can help you progress safely and more effectively regardless of what stage you are in. Certainly, you gain knowledge about how to move along the way, but there is no way to know everything. How can you be sure a movement is right if you've never done it before?

Again, this is very simplified here. Don't get me wrong. Your activity level and your goals are important, but there are other considerations that make movement and form very important. For example, many health conditions require specific safe movement principles. Musculoskeletal examples include and are not limited to degenerative changes of the spine, spinal stenosis, osteoporosis, osteoarthritis, and rheumatoid arthritis. Remember our examples in Chapter 7 that discussed common chronic conditions? Feel free to review it now. Other examples include obesity, cardiac conditions, diabetes, and neurological conditions such as Parkinson's disease. People with these conditions and others can greatly benefit from regular movement and exercise. You just need to know that many require a special focus on form so that you can move safely and effectively.

There's one very important point to add here. Make this fun for you. If you are one who likes regimen and likes to plan your exercise and activity, great. Maybe you're not quite as formal. You like to change things up and want some variety in your life. If this describes you, then please incorporate some change in your new routine. Do you like to exercise with others or do you prefer to be alone? Either way, that's okay. Design your program to your likes. Maybe you like to move with music. Excellent. I'm that person, too. Get some earbuds or headphones that allow you to do this safely. I always do more when I listen to music. It motivates me.

Remember to listen to your body, make sure you're well hydrated, and pay attention to posture and good form. I briefly mentioned the importance of balance earlier in this chapter. It's time to take a closer look at this, as it will provide another important focus for you as you design your program. And it just might be the most important one.

Chapter 11 Balancing Act

Balance training and fall prevention are critical to an adult's life. To lead an independent life and have the freedom to do what you want, you must keep your fall risk low. This is why I've devoted a whole chapter to this topic. And that's why I think balance training and fall prevention should be a part of every adult's training program.

Let's get right to it. First the bad news:

- Falls are the leading cause of injury-related death and nonfatal injuries in adults 65 and older.

- Every 13 seconds, an older adult is rushed to the hospital due to a fall.

- Each year, more than one in every four adults 65 and older falls, but fewer than half tell their doctor.

- Some 20 to 30 percent of people who fall suffer moderate to severe injuries such as lacerations, hip fractures, and head traumas.

(CDC, Home and Recreational Safety)

Now, the good news:

- Falls are not an inevitable part of aging.

- You can reduce your chance of falling.

- You have the power.

So, what are the risk factors? How can we lower our risk?

Falls are serious business and one of the major reasons an adult pursues physical therapy. Your safety depends on a lot of different factors. Effective fall prevention strategies should include medical management, environmental modifications, and, you guessed it, exercise. We'll review risk factors first and then discuss how movement and exercise can improve your balance.

Risk factors can be described as either internal or external. Internal risk factors are all about you and your health. External risk factors include what's in your environment. Let's look at internal risk factors first.

Internal risk factors include:

- Medications

- Vision

- Hearing

- Medical conditions such as orthostatic hypotension and neuropathy

- Fitness level such as poor flexibility and decreased strength

Medical management is important to address all of the above risk factors and requires visiting with your physician and specialists when asked. Be diligent with your medications, and do not make changes unless you clear it first with your doctor. Prescription medications and changes to these are often implicated in poor balance. Look at the side effects, and consult with your doctor if you suspect your medications are making you unsteady.

Have an eye exam regularly and, if you wear glasses, be sure they are appropriate for your current vision. Do you ever get light-headed or dizzy when you sit up or stand up quickly? That can be a sign of orthostatic hypotension, defined as a sudden drop in blood pressure with position changes. Dehydration may cause this as well as other underlying health conditions. Be sure to discuss this with your physician right away if you experience this. Neuropathy is a loss of sensation in your extremities and is commonly associated with diabetes. Neuropathy in your feet can cause balance issues and increase your fall risk.

Poor fitness levels are a risk factor for falls. As a result, exercise is a critical piece to improve your safety and is important for a number of reasons:

- Movement and exercise on a regular basis are critical for long-term health, fitness, and quality of life.

- Fall prevention must include movement and exercise to maximize range of motion, strength, and function.

- For those with osteoporosis or osteopenia, seek out safe bone-strengthening strategies that integrate alignment and balance techniques. Those with decreased bone density are more at risk for fractures from a fall than someone without it.

- Even if you don't have osteoporosis or osteopenia, strengthening your bones is important and can and should be done at any age.

- Know you can improve your strength and balance at any age.

External risk factors may include the following:

- Clutter

- Pets

- Poor lighting

- Hazards such as throw rugs

- Cabinets that are out of reach

- Needed handrails or other equipment

- Ill-fitting clothing, slippers, and shoes

Home modifications for external risk factors can include removing clutter from you home such as objects on the floor where you walk. Remove slippery throw rugs, and make sure your home is well lit. Install a night light for those trips to the bathroom at night. Move those frequently used dishes and cooking pans to a height that you can easily reach. Save the upper shelves for rarely used items. Install hand rails at stairs and at the entrance of your tub or shower.

Falls are all too often associated with injury. Have you had a fall in the past year? Were you hurt? Do you worry about falling? Do you feel unsteady when standing or walking? If any of your answers were yes, do you limit activities as a result? Think about this. Do you? You might and may not even realize it. Injury or not, you might have a lasting fear of falling. I call this the injury you cannot see.

Fear of falling is a lasting concern that may cause you to stop doing activities you remain able to do. In some respects, this is a valid fear as one of the best predictors of a future fall is a past fall. The more recent the fall is, the higher the chance. Most people don't like to talk about it. This may be due to embarrassment and fear of losing your independence. Thus, you ignore it. You brush it under the rug, and many times, adults don't even tell their physician about it when asked directly. If left unchecked, your fear can turn into reality. You need to address it, correct it, move, and resume your life.

Why does fear of falling matter? It may stop you from participating in your favorite activities even while you still have the capacity to do them. Legs weaken with inactivity, and inactivity leads to falls. Eventually, it can cause you to feel alone. It can even make you depressed. Don't enter this cycle of disability. Don't go down that road, friends.

I first heard about Sharon through her daughter, Lisa, who called me because she was concerned for her mother's health. "She fell a couple weeks ago and she just hasn't been the same since," Lisa said. "She was pretty banged up but thankfully had no injuries," Lisa added. "But now she's staying to herself more. She declined meeting us for dinner on Sunday," said Lisa. "She's not playing cards with her friends either. I'm worried about her." Lisa added, "At least she is using a cane now. I think that helps."

At Lisa's request, I called Sharon to meet with her to see how she was doing. She welcomed the visit. That is always a good sign. Some people refuse the help.

I met Sharon at her home. It is a fairly new manufactured home with a few steps to enter. Once inside, she lived on one floor. The home was clean and well kept. Sharon explained that she lost her balance in her living room and remembers falling toward her large picture window. She showed me where it happened. She has carpet there, and it was well lit. She denies any clutter was there when she fell. There was nothing unusual about the area. "I go by this window all the time," said Sharon. "I don't know why it happened."

What she did remember is that she wanted to avoid landing on that window at all costs and ducked. She succeeded and hit a sill that runs along the bottom of the window. She hit it so hard it broke off the wall. She has bruising on her ribs to show for it. Luckily, she didn't fracture them. Sharon has a cardiac history, and I asked her if she was lightheaded or dizzy. She said no. I then performed a physical exam, which revealed some findings that potentially could have contributed to what happened. She had tightness in her lower legs, preventing her from walking normally. This could have played a role. She had some weakness in her legs, which certainly could have contributed. There were other factors in her history that when combined with the physical findings, could have compromised her balance.

I provided some exercises for Sharon to do, and she performed them when I was there. She did well with them. I could see some relief on her face then. I asked her what she thought about the program I was setting up for her, and she was on the verge of tears. "I can do these things," she said. "Maybe I can recover from this." Sharon regained some hope. Just by welcoming me in and being honest about what happened, she opened herself up for healing–emotional healing. She had been suffering both physically and emotionally. The emotional injuries are much harder to see though her daughter saw them and acted.

Sharon was entering that disability cycle we talked about. With action and movement, she got out of that cycle. Sharon is currently doing very well and no longer needs a cane. There are no more falls, and she is out and about with family and friends routinely now.

The fear of a future fall is the injury you cannot see. The truth is, you have the power to act now to improve your health, fitness level, and your quality of life. Meet your fear head on, and do it early. Take action to improve your mobility. Keep moving.

How can we improve our balance? What are some examples of balance training? We've already made the point that movement can happen two ways. First, we have movement that we do to live our life. This starts with getting out of bed in the morning, showering, making breakfast, and perhaps going to work or a class. Maybe later, you come home and do some weeding in your garden. You sweep out the garage or do some chores inside your home. Then you make dinner. You are moving. You are changing positions, you are walking, perhaps you are walking up and down stairs, you are squatting, you are reaching. You are moving your body, and you are getting stronger from it.

Second, we have purposeful exercise or prescriptive exercise. Maybe the class you attended is a tai chi class or perhaps yoga. Wonderful. If you're not that active, you're probably wondering what you can do at home to improve your strength, mobility, and balance. If this is you, I suggest that the first thing you do is call your physician and get a referral to a local physical therapist. Maybe you know one already whom you trust to help you. Make the call. Not only is that person skilled to help you, but there is also some accountability put into play when you have to check in with someone else regularly. That can be such a huge help and may make the difference between failure and success.

Do you enjoy swimming and have access to a pool? This is an outstanding environment in which to work on your balance. When I worked as a physical therapist at a major hospital in Rochester, NY, and again for a hospital in the Finger Lakes, I taught aquatic therapy in a pool. Movement in the water has so many therapeutic benefits that make it very effective. Besides balance deficits, exercising in a pool can also help those with osteoarthritis, back pain, and degenerative conditions of the spine, including spinal stenosis and degenerative disc disease. There are three properties to water that make it the ideal environment for rehab.

Buoyancy: You are lighter in water than you are on land. When waist-deep in a pool, you are effectively 50 percent of your body weight. When chest-deep, you are 30 percent of your weight. When up to your neck in water, you're only 10 percent of your body weight. This significantly reduces joint compression in weight-bearing joints including your knees, hips, and spine. This can make movement more tolerable, and the benefits translate to your life on land.

Hydrostatic pressure. This is the pressure that the water exerts against you and all around you. It gives us feedback for our body position and allows us to work on balance training and fall prevention with minimal fear of loss of balance and injury. You can simply challenge yourself more in the water than on land.

Viscosity: Think of this as the density of the water. When you walk through it, there is resistance against you. The faster you try to walk, the more resistance this creates. This also applies to moving your limbs in the water. We can use this to progress strengthening just by using equipment that increases surface area and varying how fast you move a part through the water. This is very effective for people with joint pain anywhere in the body.

Don't forget water temperature as a factor for effective movement and exercise. Water temperature matters as the warmer it is, the more therapeutic it is. Watch out for water too warm though (higher than 90 degrees), as this can cause someone to overheat faster when they move vigorously. Temperature in the middle 80s is considered an ideal temperature for older adults.

A pool can be a wonderful way to improve your balance in a safe environment. You can't fall here. Aquatic therapy can also help you move with less pain especially if you have osteoarthritis. Water therapy and exercise can comprise or complement your current land-based activities. Many community centers and your local YMCA often provide classes in and out of the pool. Being with others can make movement even more fun as you find new friends with similar interests as yours. With so many benefits to this type of exercise, I hope you'll consider this as part of your program.

As far as balance training on land goes, some simple activities can help get you started. Below are some common exercises I routinely perform with folks in their homes to improve their balance. These are also noted in Appendix A along with strengthening and stretching exercises.

Always remember, safety first. Please consult with your physician prior to starting any new exercise program to ensure you are safe to perform these and other exercises.

Balance Training

Here are some suggestions to improve your balance.

Static Balance Training (Standing)

Perform all near the kitchen counter for safety.

- Wide to narrow BOS. Stand with feet apart and as wide as your hips. If challenging, try to hold this for up to 30 seconds. If not challenging, repeat by putting your feet closer together until they are touching. Again, try to hold this up to 30 seconds. Try to look straight ahead and not down at the floor as able. Please hold onto the counter as needed for safety.

- Eyes open to eyes closed. If you are able to stand with your feet together without holding onto the counter for 30 seconds, try doing this with your eyes closed. Try to keep your balance for up to 30 seconds as able. Perform three times as able.

- Single leg stance. Hold onto the counter while lifting up one foot off the floor. Try to keep your balance on one leg for up to 30 seconds as able. Perform three times as able.

Dynamic Balance Training (Standing)

Perform all near the kitchen counter for safety.

- Side stepping along the length of the counter. Keep your gaze straight ahead if you can do so safely, and keep your feet pointing forward (not out to the side). Start with up to five laps back and forth.

- Walking forward and backward. Hold onto the counter lightly, and walk forward and then backward. When walking forward, try to land on the heels first. When walking backward, land on the toes first. Exaggerate this if you can. This will help improve the flow of your gait.

- Sit to stand to sit. Prop up a surface of a chair with a dense pillow or foam if you have it. This makes it easier to stand and sit repeatedly for strength and balance training. Gradually lower the surface as able over time. Just be sure you can do it safely without holding your hands on the chair. Repeat 10 to 20 to 30 times as able.

———

Fall prevention gives you freedom. Fall prevention gives you independence. Don't just work on balance, think you've got this, and stop. You must continue to work on it. As we age, those physiological changes continue. They are always in play. Therefore, we must stay in play, too.

Chapter 12 You've Started—Congratulations

The key point to remember about starting an exercise program is that something is always better than nothing. Move more and sit less. Even one minute of activity is better than no activity at all. Move and keep moving. Congratulations on deciding that you are worth it.

As you decide what to do, here is my hope for you:

- I want you to make it personal.

- I want your signature on it.

- I want it to include what you can do, what challenges you, and what is meaningful for you.

- I want you to make it fun.

- I want you to keep doing it.

When all of the above happens, you will want to do it again and again. That is what matters. Consistent and regular movement makes things happen. You've likely heard the old saying, "If you don't use it, you'll lose it." Well, it's true. How you use it is up to you. Continuing what you started is the second most important thing.

You made a change. You overcame the challenges and you Got UP. Your body and your mind are reaping the benefits from your decision and your commitment. Why is this such a big deal? Because you found success. More importantly, success breeds success. This is such an important concept. If you play sports, you get this. Momentum is now on your side, and you know you can do anything you set your mind to. What a great feeling, right? Bravo.

Two of the most motivated people I know are Brenda and Bob. Both are driven, and though their goals change and evolve over time, their work ethic never waivers. This can be seen in their space at home where they exercise.

They dedicated a space in their basement to improving their fitness and quality of life. They have a rubberized floor, which is perfect for standing exercises and as the foundation for equipment. They have his and her folding exercise mats that fit their space perfectly and provide a comfortable surface for floor work, including core strengthening and stretching. They have a monitor there so Brenda can plug in a workout DVD if desired. They have a recumbent bike that both use for aerobic work. They have a punching bag, a small round floor trampoline, exercise bands, and free weights. They have the ultimate setup. Their commitment shows in each and every item.

But here's the best part. Brenda decorated the walls with prints featuring inspirational quotes and other words of encouragement. Better yet, she and her family are in every one of these. Family matters greatly to her and her husband. Some of these feature pictures taken while Brenda participated in various activities over the years such as hula-hooping on the Jersey Shore. She is surrounding herself with her goals. She props herself up with the past while she continues to look forward. With this space, she is envisioning her active future. Their space is devoted to their fit lives. This is their wellness space, and that is its sole purpose.

Please consider this if you have the space and are serious about your commitment to your active lifestyle. In northern climates, this really comes in handy during the winter months. Make it your space. Make it your sanctuary.

Your movement may change a bit over time as you progress and as you age. And that's okay. The key is movement needs to stay with you for your entire life. It is a lifestyle choice. While I know a few adults who don't like to exercise, they still do it because it works. To some of you, this whole concept of movement and exercise may sound daunting., but please listen. If you take the time to invest in yourself, you'll see results. It's that simple. It may not be easy, but it is simple. It gets easier when you see and feel the success you are having. When you have returned to the activities you enjoy and perhaps even found new ones, that, above all else, will keep you coming back.

When I repeatedly hurt my back while playing ice hockey in college, I seriously thought I'd never play hockey again. I didn't even know if I'd ever play sports again. That thought was devastating to me. When I went through physical therapy that summer of my sophomore year, I learned a lot about my back and my body. I was given another chance. No, let me rephrase that. I sought out a way to get a second chance. I worked really hard each and every day to earn that second chance. It was the only possible way I even had a chance to play sports again. And it got me there.

Just like Scott kept all his handouts as noted in Chapter 9, I have those same exercise sheets my physical therapist gave me then. That was in 1981. And what's more, I still do many of them. They helped me then, and they help me now. There is no better buy-in than something that works. Period.

As I said, I have been doing some of the same exercises I learned way back when. As I write this, I did these exercises about two hours ago. As I edit this, I also did them about two hours ago. I'm not kidding. And I will do them again tomorrow, next week, next month, and next year (God willing).

Well, you probably know me well enough now to know I like variety in my life–even a little adventure. Not much stays the same with me. Then how could I possibly do these same exercises for about 40 years? Because they work. And because I've changed them up a little over time. What you may find strange is that I didn't plan to change them up from time to time. It just happened.

I remember when the large stability balls became popular and I thought, *Well, they look like fun.* So off I went and purchased one from the local sporting goods store. I found a way to stretch and strengthen my body with this in a way that was different, effective, and challenging. I enjoyed this and still have one of these balls in my home.

I am so fortunate and grateful that my vocation has helped me personally. My patients appreciate it, too, because I talk the talk and I've walked the walk. I share everything I've learned with my own body, too. Making movement and exercise an enjoyable part of your everyday life may be easier than you think. I mentioned above my use of a stability ball from time to time. That can be a great way to strengthen your core and provide some variety into your program. Other equipment can include hand weights, cuff weights, and resistance bands as well at weighted balls and kettle bells.

Where do you exercise? Some like Brenda and Bob enjoy doing it at home. Some like going to a community center or gym to take advantage of machines and equipment. Some want to be outside as much as possible, and they design activity to their surroundings. Some like it quiet when they exercise, whereas others really need some upbeat music. It gets them fired up, and they end up moving harder than they otherwise would have. Either way is great.

There are so many activities out there that may interest you. Please consider changing things up as you continue your movement journey. Below is a list of the more popular ways people move. See if your activity is on the list. Maybe even try to find something new if that interests you and is meaningful to you.

Activities like walking, hiking, and swimming can be done with the right resources most any time. Other classes and programs may be more structured and will likely follow a schedule. The following programs are frequently offered either in person or virtually (as in via Zoom or other meeting software):

- Tai chi. An ancient Chinese system of meditative movements that can be very effective at reducing stress and improving balance.

- Yoga. A combination of mental, physical, and spiritual practices or disciplines that originated in ancient India. Although many styles exist, this posture-based physical fitness program also provides stress relief and relaxation.

- Pilates. A physical fitness system developed in the early twentieth century by Joseph Pilates, after whom it was named. It consists of low-impact flexibility, muscular strength, and endurance movements. Pilates emphasizes proper postural alignment, core strength, and muscle balance. Core strengthening has been shown to improve balance and aids in fall prevention.

- Weight training. Group strength training classes. These classes are growing in popularity. Seek out ones with the same goals as yours. Observe a class to make sure you can participate safely and confidently.

- Community classes. A wide variety of classes are offered at local recreational centers and the YMCA. Check out their offerings and again, please observe a class first to make sure it's right for you.

- Virtual classes. These have grown tremendously as a result of the COVID-19 pandemic and social distancing measures. Social distancing is not social isolation. These classes are a great way to connect with others while moving in the comfort of your own home. I continue to teach classes virtually through various organizations, and I know my participants love the opportunity to keep moving while being with others. Seek out options in your own community.

––––––––

As I said earlier, exercise is a form of movement. It is structured. It is purposeful. As you continue to move and as your program evolves, I want to share with you some principles of exercise that are simple to follow but often overlooked. Keep these in mind as you make progress on your own program.

Specificity. If you want to get better at balance, work on balance. More so, work on your balance on your feet if it is safe to do so. Otherwise, there is no other reason to work on standing balance while sitting or lying down. The only exception would be is if it is unsafe for you to do. Maybe you need more range of motion in your legs or perhaps you need more strength. Absolutely work on these things first as they will set you up for success later. Just be sure that you ultimately work specifically on your goals. If you want to get stronger, work on strengthening exercises. If you want to improve your endurance, perform cardiovascular exercise such as on a stationary bike for longer periods of time. Sounds simple, but it is often overlooked.

Overload. You need to constantly progress your program to see improvement over time. You need to overload your abilities to advance your physical condition. If you continue to work at a certain level, you will get to that level, and that's it. You continuously have to increase what you are doing and challenge yourself to get to new levels. For example, if you are performing a bicep curl with a five-pound dumbbell for 30 repetitions and never advance it, your strength will plateau at this level. To get stronger, you must increase your resistance over time. If you can perform 30 reps without fatigue at this level, add a pound or two of weight. You may not be able to perform 30 reps, but do what you can safely and then work up to 30 reps over time.

Make it enjoyable and make it yours. Keep in mind your needs and your interests may change over time. Change your movement approach right along with it. Here is where you can express yourself. No mystery here. Do what you enjoy. Mix it up. Do it with friends.

Schedule it. If you're having trouble fitting exercise into your schedule, consider it an important appointment with yourself, and mark it on your daily calendar. We often respect appointments with others more than we do with ourselves. Hard schedule it to treat your movement the same as any other commitment you make.

Make it easy on yourself. Plan your workouts for the time of day when you're most awake and energetic. If you're not a morning person, for example, don't undermine yourself by planning to exercise before work.

Remove obstacles. Plan ahead for anything that might get in the way of exercising. Do you tend to run out of time in the morning? Get your workout clothes out the night before, so you're ready to go as soon as you get up. Do you skip your evening workout if you go home first? Keep a gym bag in the car, so you can go straight from work.

Hold yourself accountable. Commit to another person. If you've got a workout partner waiting, you're less likely to skip out. Ask a friend or family member to check in on your progress. Announcing your goals to your social group (either online or in person) can also help keep you on track.

––––––––

COVID-19 has challenged how many of us move, exercise, and play sports. Organized play just stopped. Buildings closed. Pools closed. Exercise classes were cancelled. Sports stopped including professional sports for a time. What a strange time we are in. As I write this, many businesses remain closed.

We miss each other. We miss our activities. We miss the release of stress when perhaps we need it the most. Face it. We are in our homes more and just not moving much. This applies especially to older adults and retired adults. Enter Zoom and other technologies that allow us to be together, though apart. Virtual online classes have exploded in popularity, and I think they will continue to serve many adults even as businesses open back up. They can be effective, convenient, and safe for adults, and you can even get to see your friends during class. It negates barriers such as transportation and bad weather and saves time (no travel time to and from classes) with less expense. Nothing replaces face-to-face interactions, and I look forward to that returning. But know that virtual classes are a great way to keep moving and are likely here to stay.

Activity #4

Title this section *Plan.*

OK, folks, it's go time. Can you think of ways to achieve your goals? Can you come up with a plan to help you get from where you are now to where you want to be?

Perhaps you want some professional guidance from a physical therapist or occupational therapist. If that's the case, the first call should be to your physician for a consult. Express to him or her what you want to do and, as a team, create an acceptable and safe plan.

Perhaps you already have a health professional whom you consider to be a trusted resource. Make that call and discuss it further. Build your team that will potentially serve you for years to come.

How will you implement your plan? Do you want to create a devoted space to exercise in your home? Do you have any classes in mind that you'd like to attend? What kind of time commitment can you make each week, each day?

Do you have someone who might partner with you in your new journey. Find an accountability partner, and make a commitment to lift each other up.

Make the commitment, and make the choice to start now. Go ahead and make notes here for your plan. Meet you back here for the last chapter.

Chapter 13 Get Moving Now

Don't look back. Your life is ahead of you. Look forward. Look forward to the best years of your life if you let them be. The choice is yours. Isn't that great? Your life is ahead of you, and it is for you and only you to decide how to live it. How powerful is that. Part of taking ownership of where you are comes from knowing you have full control to take your life where you want to go. That jazzes me, and I hope it jazzes you, too.

Movement can take many forms. Maybe for you it's walking, swimming, golf, pickleball, or tennis. For some it's getting up from a chair and walking to the kitchen to make a meal. For others, it might be standing from a sitting position. That's okay. Some of you may not be able to move at all. But hopefully you can rely on equipment to help you move. For those of you who can move, consider it a gift, and preserve what you have at all costs. Keep moving, and you may find you can even do more than you did.

What's the right approach for you? Follow these steps to get moving and stay moving:

- Do what you enjoy. If you enjoy it, chances are you will stick with it, and that is what matters most.

- Do what is meaningful to you. Choose movement that is consistent with your goals. Remember the law of specificity: If you want to walk better, walk. If you want to sit to stand better, make sure that's part of your program. You can mix things up, but you must include what you want to improve. You wouldn't play tennis to become a better swimmer, would you?

- Do what is safe for you. Maybe dynamic balance exercises are not appropriate right now, but static ones are. Start there, and progress when safe to do so. Many modifications can be made with a good exercise program.

Movement is functional. It is necessary to live the life you want. Invest in it, and remember the returns will make you rich in terms of filling each day with activities you enjoy and with people who mean the world to you, rich in terms of living freely and independently. Wealth is freedom to do what you want. Movement is the means to your dreams.

You have the opportunity to choose how you move. Trust me when I say that in my 25 years as a physical therapist, I've spent a lot of time with folks who chose not to move. On the flip side, I've seen a lot of folks who do move and the results show.

The oldest patient I have ever treated was 102 years young. I met her when I was working at a sports medicine clinic in Upstate New York. According to her prescription from her orthopedic physician, she was coming to see me for arthritis in her left knee. Overall, she was in good health, and she had a great sense of humor. She once approached the skeleton hanging in our clinic and asked, "What happened to you?" I laughed and said, "He didn't do his home exercise program." She responded, "Oh my, I better do mine."

She walked in unassisted, with no device. Her walking speed was about the same as mine (only about 60 years separated us). She had been having increased pain in that knee recently and wanted to decrease her pain and tolerate trips to the store more comfortably. She wanted to keep her independence. That is what really was at stake here. Upon evaluation, her knee motion was limited, and muscles in her leg were tight and weaker than they should be. Eight visits later, I discharged her with all her goals met. She was motivated to get better and complied with everything I asked her to do. (She saw what happened if she didn't.) Her prescriptive exercise program included stretching and strengthening exercises and some balance training as well. She is one of those patients a therapist never forgets.

Preserving your ability to move is the most important thing you can do for yourself. Period. Think of what makes a happy and fulfilling life for you. Remember that every time you move, every time you exercise, you are putting money in your body bank. You are building up your savings to do the things you want to do. You are investing in your body to make your next years your best years. I've heard it described a number of ways, but please consider this.

I propose that we have grand pillars, set on a solid foundation, that make a life and allow us to survive and thrive from beginning to end. And, you bet, movement is the foundation for all of the pillars. Built atop this foundation are the pillars: nutrition, connection, happiness, and gratitude.

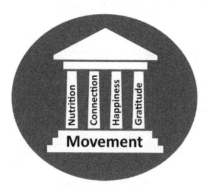

Movement allows the other parts of your life to happen and even thrive. Movement is the foundation that lifts all the others up. Movement paves the way for you to shop healthy and, therefore, eat healthy. Movement allows you to go out of your home and be with others, to connect with others. Movement allows you to laugh with others, to work, to have fun, to be happy. For example, movement allows me to play golf, which is fun most of the time. I'm working on it. When you move and have all these other aspects of your life in your hands, how can you not be grateful? Movement makes all the pillars come to life.

I challenge you to move, even if you can't imagine how you will. Find a way, and watch the other facets of your life–your pillars–come to life. I once treated a woman, Anne, with post-polio syndrome, a condition that affects polio survivors many years after recovery from the polio virus. The most common symptoms include progressive muscle weakness, fatigue, and a decrease in muscle size (called muscle atrophy). Pain from joint deterioration and deformities such as scoliosis are common. Anne was in her 70s and, well, she had it tough. Luckily, she was even tougher.

Though she couldn't walk due to post-polio syndrome, she was as mobile as she could be. She had a ceiling track system in her small home to take her from bed to wheelchair and bedroom to bathroom. Out of the home, she used a wheelchair and used her arms to propel herself to her vehicle. She had a lift to get her and her wheelchair into her vehicle. Once in the driver's seat, she used hand controls so she could drive and go to the store. She could visit with friends. Her condition did not stop her. Though she couldn't walk, she found a way to move. She moved every day and arguably had a very good quality of life as a result. Anne was grateful for what she could do.

She inspired me more than she knew. I remember belonging to the local YMCA at the time when I was treating her. I worked out a couple of days a week to keep in shape for hockey season. I loved the stepper back then, and I remember pounding those steps as hard as I could. I wouldn't do it now because of the impact. But hey, I loved that thing. Often, I thought of Anne when I was on it. I thought that even though that woman worked so hard, she would never be able to do this, much less walk. I felt sadness for her. And here I was, healthy and able to change my condition. I was so grateful that I could do this. I was so grateful I could make my body stronger so I could enjoy my life, my sports. Someone asked me why I worked out so hard. I replied, "Because I can."

I am so passionate about movement that I really feel it's a crime not to move when physically you can. Again, many are unable to move or walk due to other reasons–injuries and disease that cannot be reversed. I'm not talking about them. I am talking about you–the ones who can move but choose not to. This choice in midlife will lead to pain and disability. And when you are too far gone, physicians, therapists, and, heck, even your orthopedic surgeon won't be able to save you. As therapists, we can't magically take you back to where you were 20 years ago with a month of home visits twice per week. It just can't happen.

Let me paint a clearer picture. Stop moving, and you will become so stiff and weak that you will be unable to reach your feet to put on your socks and shoes. Your shoes will be slip-on only or may have elastic laces in place that don't require any tying from you. You will be sitting in an electric lift chair probably about 80 to 90 percent of the day and press the button to raise the chair up high because you can't stand from a chair at normal height. Your only trip will be to the bathroom and maybe the kitchen to fix a quick meal. Oh, and you will eventually sleep in that very same chair because it is too difficult to get in and out of bed. Don't believe me? When I worked in homecare, these folks were easily the majority of my patients.

At this point, who is doing the grocery shopping for you? Who is doing your laundry? Who is cleaning and maintaining your home? Who is feeding your cats or your dog? Who is transporting you to your doctor's visits? Who is coming to see you to visit and socialize? Do you put them to work when they do?

It's a vicious circle. When you stay home, you are less active. And the less you move, the weaker you become. You become stiffer, and your balance becomes more compromised, putting you at risk for falls. In isolation, which is truly what this becomes, you become less happy, and depression soon follows. The less you move, the more frail you become. Please, friends, don't go down the road of despair when the solution is right in front of you to grasp.

This couldn't be more important during our COVID-19 pandemic. We are forced into isolation a number of ways. First, we are told to stay home as that is our safest place. Second, even when we can leave our home, we don't want to because we risk contracting this disease. This is a challenge our lifetime has never seen. And we must, we must find ways to move. I have never cleaned my house more. I'm creating projects just to move. When I do a lot of writing in one day, I take a lot of breaks, usually to wash some dishes or put a load of laundry in or maybe sweep the lanai. I actually leave these little chores for myself, because I know I'll need to get up and move from time to time. Save some activities and projects for times like these. Call it busy work. Call it healthy habits. It works. Move, folks. Please move.

And keep moving. Can you see what's at stake here? We are talking about how you spend every minute of every day for the rest of your life. Movement is the means to your dreams.

Your dreams lie in the plan you just created for yourself while reading this book. Reread your plan. Get inspired about what you just created for yourself. Do you have any new ideas? Just write them down. You may not pursue everything you thought about, and that's okay. I'd actually be surprised if you did. The beauty of it is this—you've created a way to start. It's a way to get moving that is meaningful to you. Good job.

Please take action and do it now. Make the call and share with your physician your new plan. Put your new life in *motion* (pun intended). Share it with me if you like. I would love to know your plan, and I hope you'll reach out to me if you need any assistance.

Email me at movementsolutions55@gmail.com. The rest of my contact information is noted in later pages of this book. Let's be a team. Let's be here for each other. Let's be stronger together. Investigate classes in your community. Start a new walking club in your neighborhood. Join my free Living Well Academy (details can be found later in this book). Watch my videos, and find some exercises that help you reach your goals. You have so many options. Use your new plan as a springboard to a healthier future. I look forward to hearing about your success.

Sheri Salata, author of *The Beautiful No*, gets it. Her book is about her transcendence in middle age so she can live a more meaningful life. She learned how important movement and exercise are. Better late than never. "If you don't find a way to make movement your friend," said Salata, "not only will you never have the body of your dreams, your reduced quality of life may make your life unlivable."

Salata goes on to say, "Movement is one of the secret superpowers that enable you to extend your dreaming life. Movement is a privilege, a joy, even a kind of a miracle. Our bodies are the vessels for our dreams." (Salata, The Beautiful No)

Amen, sister.

So many of you over 50 think you're too old to try new things. You think it's too late. You think you're not capable of achieving an active and vibrant life. Now you know better. Now you know it's only you who you need to convince. What the old programming is telling you is just not true. What's really true is that you can always make your next years your best years.

Use movement to jumpstart your own transcendence. Have you thought about how you want to spend your next years? Are you on the cusp of a life change and looking for a way to get started? Start it with you. Start with movement, and watch the other aspects of your life grow in ways that will astound you.

Get up. Wear your superpower cape, and work that miracle. Defy aging with movement. A sedentary life is not the answer. Movement is. If you're ready to start moving, trust your physician and your other healthcare professionals, and get the guidance you need to get started. Just start and trust in the miracle of movement to raise your life to levels not yet seen. Keep depositing good health into your account, and watch your reserves grow. It will pay off.

Health is wealth. You have the power to make your next years your best years. Start now. And keep moving.

Appendix A: Prescriptive Exercise

Please see the following for details on how to perform each of the strengthening exercises, stretching exercises, and balance training. Within each group, exercises are listed in alphabetical order except for balance training where the progression is from static to dynamic training. Please note that supine means to lay on your back.

Strengthening Exercises

Ankle pumps (supine). Move both ankles at the same time to lift up forefeet, and then point the feet. Repeat up to 10 times, and progress to 30 reps slowly, over time.

Bicep curl (seated). Start with your arms straight and at your side. Face your palms forward, and bend both elbows at the same time. Bend as far as you can comfortably, and then straighten both elbows out. Repeat up to 10 times, and progress to 30 reps slowly, over time.

Clam (seated). Sit at the edge of your chair with your feet flat on the floor and side by side. With your knees also touching, wrap a light resistance band around your thighs (just above your knees). Secure with a single knot, and hold it with one hand. Then, while holding the band securely, move both knees out to the side and then slowly back into starting position. Perform up to 10 repetitions, and progress to 30 reps slowly, over time.

Clam (supine). Lay on your back with your knees bent and your feet flat on the floor or mat. As in the seated exercise, wrap a light resistance band around your thighs (just above your knees). Secure with a knot or use a continuous band that requires you to place each foot inside it, and then slide it up into position. Then, move both knees out to the side and then slowly back into starting position. Perform up to 10 repetitions, and progress to 30 reps slowly, over time.

Glut sets (supine). Squeeze your buttocks together, hold three seconds, and release. Perform up to 10 times, and progress to 30 reps slowly, over time. Breathe normally.

Heel raises (seated). Raise both heels off the floor at the same time, and then slowly lower. Perform up to 10 times, and progress to 30 reps slowly, over time.

Heel/toe raises (standing). Perform at the kitchen counter, and use as a touch point for safety. Rock back and forth by raising up on your toes, and then rock back and try to lift the toes. Perform up to 10 times each way, and progress to 30 reps slowly, over time.

Heel slides (supine). Slowly slide one heel up toward your buttock, bending your knee as much as you can comfortably. Then lower all the way back down. Perform up to 10 times with each leg, and progress to 30 reps slowly, over time. Don't alternate legs for this one.

Hip abduction (standing). Perform at the kitchen counter for safety, and hold on as needed. Lift one leg out to the side. Keep feet parallel to each other, and slowly lower back down. Perform up to 10 times with each leg, and progress to 30 reps slowly, over time. Don't alternate legs for this one. Stand up tall.

Hip extension (standing). Perform at the kitchen counter for safety, and hold on as needed. Lift one leg behind you, keeping this knee as straight as you can. Return to starting position. Perform up to 10 times with each leg, and progress to 30 reps slowly, over time. Don't alternate legs for this one. Stand up tall. (Don't lean forward).

Kickouts (seated). Straighten one knee by raising this foot off the floor. Then lower your foot back to starting position. Perform up to 10 reps with each leg (don't alternate), and work up to 30 reps as able over time.

Marches (seated). Sit in a chair, lift one knee up toward the ceiling, and then lower. Repeat with the other leg, and continue in an alternating pattern. Perform up to 10 times with each leg, and progress to 30 reps slowly, over time.

Marches (standing). Perform at the kitchen counter for safety, and hold on as needed. Lift one knee up toward the ceiling, and then lower. Repeat with the other leg, and continue in an alternating pattern. Perform up to 10 times with each leg, and progress to 30 reps slowly, over time.

Quad sets (supine). With both legs straight, tighten your thigh muscles, and press your knees down to the floor or mat. Hold for three seconds, and release. Perform up to 10 times, and progress to 30 reps slowly, over time. Breathe normally.

Pelvic tilts (supine). Bend both knees, and rest your arms at your sides. Pull in your belly button to your spine. Then release. Try not to press down with your feet. Let your abdominals do the work here. Perform up to 10 times, and progress to 30 reps slowly, over time.

Planks (prone or facing floor/mat). Place your hands on a mat with your wrists under your shoulders. Rise up, and support yourself with your hands and feet, and make a straight line with your body, head to feet. Keep your head in neutral. Hold for five seconds, and then lower down or place your knees on a mat for rest. Attempt three to five repetitions. Breathe normally.

Planks (prone to side-lying). Get into a prone position as above, and then rotate your body to the right, lifting your right hand off the mat, and stop when your body is facing right with your right arm up in the air toward the ceiling. Hold three to five seconds, and return to prone plank. Repeat to the left as above. Let your feet roll and be on their side when you turn. This is advanced and should only be performed after performing the above planks consistently with good form. Breathe normally.

Punches (seated). Press one arm into the air in front of you, and then return to starting position. Repeat with the other arm. Perform by alternating your arms up to 10 times each arm, and progress to 30 reps slowly, over time.

Rows (seated). Sit at the edge of a chair and extend arms out straight in front of you (thumbs toward the ceiling). Bring both arms behind you as if to row. Do not hike up your shoulders. Your focus should be on squeezing your shoulder blades together versus how far back your elbows move. Hold three seconds, and return to starting position. Perform up to 10 times, and progress to 30 reps slowly, over time.

Squats (standing). Stand in front of a chair, or hold onto the kitchen counter as needed for safety. Act as if you are going to sit down, but don't. Only bend your knees and hips slightly before rising back up into standing.

Keep your knees behind your toes. Hold onto the counter as needed for balance. Perform up to 10 times, and progress to 30 reps slowly, over time.

Straight leg raise (supine). Bend one knee, and keep the other knee straight. Lift the straight leg no higher than the other knee. Slowly lower down to starting position. Perform up to 10 times, and progress to 30 reps slowly, over time. Breathe normally.

Tabletop foot taps (supine). Lie on your back with your knees bent and your feet flat on the floor or mat. Arms are resting on the mat at your sides. Keeping your trunk in neutral spine, raise one leg at a time so your knees are over your hips and your knees are bent 90 degrees. Your shins should be parallel to the floor. From here, tap each foot onto the mat, starting with the right and alternating legs. Keep a neutral spine throughout. Perform 5 to 10 reps each leg, and work up to 30 reps with each leg over time as able. Breathe normally.

———

A word about neutral spine. It is the natural position of your spine. We all have natural curves, and this is your neutral spine. You can help find it by performing the pelvic tilts. For example, when lying supine, first flatten your back against the mat, and then pull it away from the mat as far as you can. Then release the latter position, and let your back relax in between those two positions. This is your neutral spine.

All of the above exercises can be done seated, standing (especially by a kitchen counter for safety), or lying down. A mat on the floor is ideal, but if that is too difficult for you, a firm bed is fine. If you can easily get down to the floor and rise back up, consider a thick mat to put on the floor or carpet for a well-supported surface. Many exercises noted for supine position can also be done reclined if there is no other alternative.

Stretching Exercises

Calf stretch (standing). Hold onto the kitchen counter for safety. Slide one foot back, and keep that foot pointing forward and that knee straight. Bend the knee of the other leg in front of you, and lunge forward until a gentle stretch is felt in the calf of the back leg. Hold up to 30 seconds as able, and perform three reps each leg. You may repeat with the same leg, or alternate legs.

Hamstring stretch (seated). Sit at the edge of a chair. Place one heel on the floor out in front of you, so this knee is straight. Slowly lean forward at the hips (don't round your back) until a gentle stretch is felt behind this leg. Hold up to 30 seconds as able, and perform three reps with each leg. You may repeat with the same leg, or alternate legs.

Knee to chest stretch (supine) . Bring one knee up toward your chest, and help it with your arms as able. Hold for a gentle stretch for 10 to 30 seconds as able. Then lower. Repeat with the other leg, and alternate legs for three reps each.

Balance Training

Static Balance Training (Standing)

Hold onto a kitchen counter as needed for safety.

Wide to narrow BOS. Stand with your feet apart and as wide as your hips. If challenging, try to hold this for up to 30 seconds. If not challenging, repeat by putting your feet closer together until they are touching. Again, try to hold this up to 30 seconds. Try to look straight ahead and not down at the floor as able. Please hold onto the counter as needed for safety.

Eyes open to eyes closed. If you are able to stand with your feet together for 30 seconds without holding onto a counter as above, try doing this with your eyes closed. Try to keep your balance for up to 30 seconds as able. Perform three times as able.

Single leg stance. Hold onto a counter while lifting up one foot off the floor. Try to keep your balance on one leg for up to 30 seconds as able. Perform three times as able.

Dynamic Balance Training (Standing)

Hold onto a kitchen counter as needed for safety.

Side stepping along the length of the counter. Keep your gaze straight ahead if you can do so safely, and keep your feet pointing forward (not out to the side). Start with up to five laps back and forth.

Walking forward and backward. Hold onto a counter lightly, and walk forward and then backward. When walking forward, try to land on the heels first. When walking backward, land on your toes first. Exaggerate this if you can. This will help improve the flow of your gait.

Sit to stand to sit. Prop up a surface of a chair with a dense pillow or foam if available to make it easier to stand and sit repeatedly for strength and balance training. Gradually lower the surface as able, as long as you can safely do it without holding on with your hands on the chair. Repeat 10 to 20 to 30 times as able.

Appendix B: Exercise Intensity

Let's now think about how intense our movement should be. You most certainly want it effective and yet safe. There are a number of ways to assess this. Intensity can be thought of in three levels:

- Low-intensity activity. You can easily talk in full sentences or sing.

- Moderate intensity. You can speak in full sentences but not sing.

- Vigorous intensity. You are too breathless to speak in full sentences.

For the general population, aiming for moderate-intensity exercise is thought to be sufficient to improve your overall health. For me, when treating older adults in the rehabilitation setting, this moderate intensity is actually the highest level I will use. That is to say, with anyone I work with over 55, if you cannot speak a full sentence because you are too breathless, you need to slow it down. You should always be able to speak a full sentence without limitation. You should breathe a little heavier than normal but not be out of breath. Your body should feel warmer as you move but not overheated or sweating profusely. This is especially important for our sedentary population.

The above is a simple way to monitor intensity. Research provides some other ways we can assess physical activity intensity. Here, we will discuss the Borg rating of perceived exertion (RPE) and target heart rate guidelines.

Borg Rating of Perceived Exertion (RPE)

According to the Centers for Disease Control and Prevention, perceived exertion is how hard you feel like your body is working. It is based on the physical sensations a person experiences during physical activity, including increased heart rate, increased respiration or breathing rate, increased sweating, and muscle fatigue. Although this is a subjective measure, your exertion rating, based on a 6 to 20 rating scale, may provide a fairly good estimate of your actual heart rate during physical activity. (CDC, Physical Activity/Exertion)

You can rate your perceived exertion as noted in the following table. For example, a rating of 6 implies no exertion. A 20 rating perceives a maximal exertion of effort. Practitioners generally agree that perceived exertion ratings between 12 to 14 on the Borg Scale suggests that physical activity is being performed at a moderate level of intensity.

To use the Borg Scale yourself, assign numbers based on how you feel at any given time. Self-monitoring how hard your body is working can help you adjust the intensity of the activity by speeding up or slowing down your movements.

Rating	Perceived Exertion
6	No exertion
7	Extremely light
8	
9	Very light
10	
11	Light
12	
13	Somewhat hard
14	
15	Hard
16	
17	Very hard
18	
19	Extremely hard
20	Maximal exertion

A high correlation exists between a person's perceived exertion rating times 10 and the actual heart rate during physical activity. Your exertion rating may provide a fairly good estimate of the actual heart rate during activity. For example, if your RPE is 12, then 12 x 10 = 120, so your heart rate should be approximately 120 beats per minute. Note that this calculation is only an approximation of heart rate, and the actual heart rate can vary quite a bit, depending on age and physical condition. The Borg RPE is also the preferred method to assess intensity among those individuals who take medications that affect heart rate. For example, taking a beta blocker medication for managing abnormal heart rhythms stabilizes your heart rate regardless of your activity level. In this case, taking your pulse to determine your heart rate is not a reliable indicator of exertion.

Target Heart Rate

For moderate-intensity physical activity, your target heart rate should be between 64 and 76 percent of your maximum heart rate, according to the Centers for Disease Control and Prevention. (CDC, Physical Activity/Heart Rate)

You can estimate your maximum heart rate based on your age. To estimate your maximum age-related heart rate, subtract your age from 220. For example, for a 50-year-old person, the estimated maximum age-related heart rate would be calculated as 220–50 years = 170 beats per minute (bpm). The 64 percent level would be 170 x 0.64 = 109 bpm, and the 76 percent level would be 170 x 0.76 = 129 bpm.

This shows that moderate-intensity physical activity for a 50-year-old person will require that the heart rate remains between 109 and 129 bpm during physical activity.

Many devices and pieces of equipment will calculate your heart rate for you. I often use a device called a pulse oximeter to check my patient's pulse, and I even own one of these personally. This device measures both heart rate and the percent of oxygen in your blood. Most commonly, a sensor is applied to a thin part of a person's body, typically a fingertip. Wavelengths of light pass through the body part to help measure these parameters due to the pulsing of arterial blood. Though I find this very helpful when working with older adults, there are cases when the pulse reading is unreliable. For example, it is not considered accurate if someone has an irregular heartbeat such as that with a condition called atrial fibrillation. You then should resort to manually taking your pulse.

Not everyone has this kind of equipment, but everyone can manually take his or her pulse. To check your pulse, I recommend using the wrist. You can feel the radial pulse on the artery of the wrist in line with the thumb. Place the tips of the index and middle fingers over the artery and press lightly. This is important, because pressing too hard alters your normal rhythm. Do not use the thumb. Take a full 60-second count of the heartbeats, or take a 30-second count and multiply by two. Start the count on a beat, which is counted as zero. For example, if this number falls between 109 and 129 bpm in the case of a 50-year-old person, he or she is active within the target range for moderate-intensity activity.

I check vital signs including pulse and blood pressure frequently for my patients at the start of every visit. It helps me know if it's safe for patients to exercise, especially when they have compromising medical conditions. I can also see trends and know instantly if a reading is not the patient's norm. I use an oxygen saturation rate of at least 90 percent to decide if patients should exercise or not. If their reading is under 90 percent, I will likely recheck it a few times and ask if he or she has any symptoms such as shortness of breath or dizziness. If this reading continues, I do not proceed with exercise and likely alert the patient's physician. Please consult with your own physician if you have any questions related to this.

———

Oxygen saturation rate can also be helpful as it relates to COVID-19. Drops in oxygen saturation can indicate something else is going on, even when the patient otherwise feels fine. If something is going on, this can get valuable treatment started sooner. Units are available to purchase online for as little as $30.

Pulse Oximeter in Use

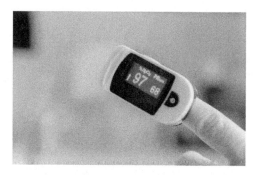

(iStockphoto.com)

Appendix C: Posture

There is something very important to you as you live your life and move, and that is posture. What is posture and why is it so important? Posture is body position. It is one part of your body and its relationship to another part of your body. It constitutes joint positions, angles, soft tissue length, and tension among and between structures. It's really quite fascinating. Let's take a further look and relate it to your everyday activities. Trust me. It's worth it.

Posture can be in either a static state or a dynamic state. Static posture means there is limited to no movement of your body. Sitting, for example, is considered a static posture. Dynamic posture is characterized by constant motion. An example of this includes walking or even lifting an object off the floor. You are likely in a seated position right now. Are you sitting upright, or have you slid down lower or slouched in your chair? Is your chair hard or soft? Is it high or low? Are your feet on the floor, or are you standing up? Perhaps you have a standing desk, so you don't have to sit so often. Are you sitting on a stability ball? Some people do.

Posture matters. It matters because when it's not right, you can hurt. If you continue to ignore the signs, then damage can occur. Pain is one of the main reasons people see a physical therapist. It is the most common diagnosis I have seen on a prescription throughout my entire career. And often, it is due to poor posture. The good news is if we catch poor posture early enough, we can correct it with minimal to no damage. With a thorough evaluation, we can identify the cause of pain and start to correct it right away. It's one of the easiest symptoms to treat and starts with following some pretty basic rules.

Here they are:

Keep the natural curves in your spine. We all have natural curves in our spine. At the neck, there is an inward curve. As we travel lower, the thoracic spine has an outward curve. Keep travelling down, and the lumbar spine has an inward curve, followed by an outward curve made by the sacrum. We all have different size curves that can change as you age. You may have a larger lumbar curve than someone else. Someone may have what's called a flat back at the lumbar levels, which means there is little to no curve. We're all different., but we can respect our own curves and try to keep these curves as close to normal as possible during our daily activities. This applies to both static and dynamic posture.

Side View of the Spine Facing to the Right

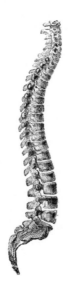

(iStockphoto.com)

Don't slouch. By this I mean don't reverse your lumbar curve. Slouching causes you to have an outward curve at the lumbar spine, not the inward curve you had at birth. This causes significant stress on soft tissue including tendons and ligaments. You see, they need to lengthen under tension to keep you in this position, and this causes pain and injury if performed long enough. How can you correct this? Sit with good lumbar support that fills the gap between your chair and your lumbar spine. This helps to passively get you back to your natural curves. The beauty of this is that correction here helps your entire spine. It helps restore your natural spinal curves from the bottom to the top. The next item can also help you avoid slouching.

Proper Posture While Seated

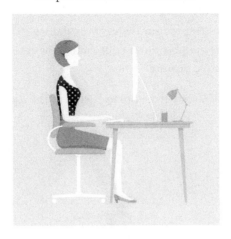

(iStockphoto.com)

Keep your hips slightly higher than your knees–this one is often overlooked. When seated, see how high your hips are relative to your knees. It's hard to see this yourself, so you may need a mirror or someone else to view this accurately. Why is this important? When your hips are higher, this facilitates your low back to be in its more natural curve. The deeper or lower your hips are, the more your lumbar spine has to flex (bend forward) to accommodate this.

Avoid extreme positions in your joints. Each joint has what we call an end range. For example, look at your wrist. You can bend your wrist, so the palm gets closer to your forearm, or you can move it the other way. When you go as far as you can in both directions, that's your end range. It is best not to statically hold your wrist at an end range for an extended length of time or even do work here. This can often occur while sitting at your computer or laptop. Take a look at your posture. Is your wrist near end range, or is it more in the middle? Being in the middle is best, as illustrated. Avoid end-range positions of your joints to minimize stress and tension on these structures.

Proper posture helps decrease pain as well as damage to joints and soft tissue, and that's a great investment to make for your body over the long term.

Appendix D: Exercise Session Structure

You might be wondering how to structure the recommended activities into in a single session. I recommend the following order.

Aerobic

Perform this first. Warm up with dynamic active movements that warm the muscles you'll be using. The simplest activity here is walking. If space is limited, you can perform other activities sitting or standing such as marches, heel raises, or arm swings. Another alternative is something called a floor bike that you can buy and place on the floor in front of a sturdy chair. Here you can place your feet on the pedals and have it work just like a stationary bicycle. The beauty is its portability, and very little space is needed.

You can also consider a dynamic warmup to be a slower, easier version of the upcoming exercises, too. For example, if you're going to run, warm up with walking. If you are performing an aerobic activity in your session, this is a great start.

Exercise or Sporting Activity

This includes the exercises, particularly strengthening exercises, as noted previously. When you're more active, this may include running or a sport such as golf or pickleball.

Cooldown and Stretching

Depending on your activity or workout, it's important to take a few minutes to cool down and allow your heart rate to return to its resting rate. This might be a short walk, for example. A cooldown should also include some gentle stretches, which can also help prevent soreness and injuries. Static stretches of up to 30 seconds are very effective and should always be done after an activity, never before. Stretches are included in your exercise prescription and are noted as such in Appendix A.

———

Keeping all this in mind, your exercise session might look like this:

- Warmup activity. Walk or use floor bike for 5 to 10 minutes.

- Exercise or sporting activity. Perform seated or standing strengthening exercises. Core and balance training would be appropriate here, too, or perform your activity or sport.

- Cooldown activity. Slow your movement down for a few minutes to help normalize your heart rate. Don't just stop a vigorous activity suddenly. You risk decreased blood flow to the brain and dizziness. Walk around slowly to cool down. Then, once your heart rate has normalized, stretch with static holds as instructed for maximal effectiveness.

Bibliography

Alexander, Nancy. *An Unlikely Gift: Finding Inspiration Caring for My Father with Dementia.* Canandaigua: Aging Well Now, 2018.

American Diabetes Association (ADA). "Get and Stay Fit." Accessed November 24, 2020. https://www.diabetes.org/exercise-and-type-1.

Centers for Disease Control and Prevention. "Arthritis." Accessed November 24, 2020. https://www.cdc.gov/arthritis/basics/osteoarthritis.htm.

Centers for Disease Control and Prevention. "Coronavirus Disease 2019 (COVID-19)." Accessed November 24, 2020. https://www.cdc.gov/coronavirus/2019-ncov/symptoms-testing/symptoms.html.

Centers for Disease Control and Prevention. "Home and Recreational Safety." Accessed November 25, 2020. https://www.cdc.gov/homeandrecreationalsafety/falls/adultfalls.html

Centers for Disease Control and Prevention. "National Center for Health Statistics." Accessed November 24, 2020. https://www.cdc.gov/nchs/fastats/alzheimers.htm.

Centers for Disease Control and Prevention. "Physical Activity/Exertion." Accessed November 24, 2020. https://www.cdc.gov/physicalactivity/basics/measuring/exertion.htm.

Centers for Disease Control and Prevention. "Physical Activity/Heart Rate." Accessed November 24, 2020. https://www.cdc.gov/physicalactivity/basics/measuring/heartrate.htm.

Cure Alzheimer's Fund. "Dementia." Accessed November 25, 2020. https://curealz.org/the-disease/dementia/.

Friedman, Susan M., MD, MPH. "A Lifestyle Medicine Approach to COVID-19." Accessed November 25, 2020. https://www.rochesterlifestylemedicine.com/author/susan-friedman/.

Harvard Health Letter. "Exercise benefits the heart even when it doesn't shrink the waistline." July 2012. Accessed November 25, 2020. https://www.health.harvard.edu/press_releases/exercise-benefits-the-heart-even-when-it-doesnt-shrink-the-waistline.

Harvard Health Letter. "Exercise can add years to your life." February 2013. Accessed November 25, 2020. https://www.health.harvard.edu/staying-healthy/exercise-can-add-years-to-your-life.

Levine, Hallie. "5 Ways to Boost Your Immune System." Updated May 5, 2020. Accessed November 25, 2020. https://www.aarp.org/health/healthy-living/info-2020/boosting-immune-response.html.

Merriam-Webster.com dictionary. "Ageism." Accessed November 25, 2020. https://www.merriam-webster.com/dictionary/ageism.

Merriam-Webster.com dictionary. "Physical Therapy." Accessed November 25, 2020. https://www.merriam-webster.com/dictionary/physical%20therapy.

Merriam-Webster.com dictionary. "Rehabilitation." Accessed November 25, 2020. https://www.merriam-webster.com/dictionary/rehabilitation.

National Institutes of Health (NIH). "National Institute on Aging (NIA)." Accessed November 24, 2020. https://www.nia.nih.gov/about/aging-strategic-directions-research/goal-biology-impact.

National Osteoporosis Foundation (NOF). "What is Osteoporosis and What Causes It?" Accessed November 24, 2020. https://www.nof.org/patients/what-is-osteoporosis/.

Reynolds, Gretchen. "Which Type of Exercise Is Best for the Brain?" The New York Times. February 17, 2016. https://well.blogs.nytimes.com/2016/02/17/which-type-of-exercise-is-best-for-the-brain/.

Salata, Sheri. "The Beautiful No." New York: HarperCollins Publishers, 2019.

Tolppanen, Anna-Maija, et al. "Leisure-time physical activity from mid- to late life, body mass index, and risk of dementia." Alzheimer's & Dementia Volume 11, Issue 4. (April 2014) https://alz-journals.onlinelibrary.wiley.com/doi/10.1016/j.jalz.2014.01.008.

U.S. Department of Education, "Title IX and Sex Discrimination." Accessed November 25, 2020. https://www2.ed.gov/about/offices/list/ocr/docs/tix_dis.html.

U.S. Department of Health and Human Services. "Physical Activity Guidelines for Americans, 2nd edition." Accessed November 25, 2020. https://health.gov/sites/default/files/2019-09/Physical_Activity_Guidelines_2nd_edition.pdf).

World Health Organization. "Healthy Ageing." Accessed November 25, 2020. https://www.who.int/ageing/ageism/en/.

About the Author

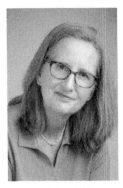

Nancy Alexander is a licensed physical therapist with a passion to serve adults over 50 to help make their next years their best years. Nancy has treated thousands of patients over her 25-year career in many different settings. She holds numerous specialist certifications including Certified Strength and Conditioning Specialist with the National Strength and Conditioning Association, Senior Fitness Specialist with the American Council on Exercise, and Licensed Buff Bones® Instructor. Over 50 herself, her mission is to provide hope and guidance to others to help them feel better, move better, and live better.

Nancy owns Professional Movement Solutions, LLC, where she works privately with adults and teaches specialized fitness classes both in person and virtually. Her online classes are increasingly popular with participants enrolled from across the country. She holds a degree from the University of Buffalo in Physical Therapy and from SUNY College at Oswego in English/Writing Arts. She regularly serves an engaged community via her Living Well Academy blog. She is a published author and popular speaker and is actively engaged in organizations mentoring others. Before gaining her physical therapy degree in her 30s, Nancy worked as a marketing and public relations professional at major firms in New York City and Rochester, NY.

Nancy cared for her father for 18 years after her mother died, which inspired her to write a memoir about their relationship and journey titled, *An Unlikely Gift: Finding Inspiration Caring for My Father with Dementia.* This was Nancy's first book and was published in September 2018.

A self-described athlete, Nancy continues to stay active playing golf, pickleball, biking, and exercising regularly. While managing her own injuries along the way, she's had to make some choices, but stopping isn't one of them.

The Living Well Academy

Keep Moving with Free Membership to The Living Well Academy

Make your next years your best years by joining our Living Well Academy. If you agree that movement is the foundation of a meaningful and fulfilling life and you want to be part of a caring and vibrant community, this is the place for you. This new educational platform from Professional Movement Solutions will help you find the information, resources, and tools you need to improve your health, fitness level, and quality of life.

There is nothing to buy. All we offer is educational and supportive information to help you live a better life. It's not just a membership. It's a community. Currently at over 500 members, we learn together, share our stories, and support each other to feel better, move better, and live better.

New classes, courses, and workshops are added all year long, so you'll want to stay up to date. Most programs will remain online, but know that live and in-person events will also be offered once safe to do so.

What you'll get with your free membership:

- Monthly newsletter. Gain education and inspiration to help keep you on track with your fitness goals.

- Video library. Gain access to a collection of videos to help you learn how to move safely and more effectively. More exercises are added regularly, and many of the exercises featured in this book are available now to view.

- Expert education. Expect knowledge and information from a licensed and certified professional.

- Supportive community. Learn by reading and listening to stories of real people overcoming their challenges and living their best life as featured in our Living Well Academy blog.

- Valuable discounts. Save on workshops and courses both virtually and in-person when safe to do so.

Bonus Offer

If you sign up now, you'll also receive my new free e-book, *7 Ways to Improve Back Pain*. This second-edition book (in PDF format) features new information and guidance and is for anyone who experiences back pain that impacts everyday life. Here you will learn simple steps you can take today to help decrease and even eliminate back pain. Are you ready to feel better now? Sign up now.

Join the Living Well Academy now and get your free e-book immediately by visiting https://www.prosolutions55.com/living-well-academy/.

Come join us… because, truly, the best is yet to come.

Keep moving,

Nancy

Notes